Springer Series in Statistics

Springer

New York
Berlin
Heidelberg
Hong Kong
London
Milan
Paris
Tokyo

Springer Series in Statistics

(continued after index)

S. Huet
A. Bouvier
M.-A. Poursat
E. Jolivet

Statistical Tools for Nonlinear Regression

A Practical Guide With S-PLUS and R Examples

Second Edition

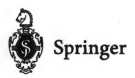

Springer

S. Huet
A. Bouvier
E. Jolivet
Laboratoire de Biométrie
INRA
78352 Jouy-en-Josas Cedex
France

M.-A. Poursat
Laboratoire de Mathématiques
Université Paris-Sud
91405 Orsay Cedex
France

Library of Congress Cataloging-in-Publication Data
Huet, S. (Sylvie)
    Statistical tools for nonlinear regression : a practical guide with S-PLUS and R
examples / Sylvie Huet, Annie Bouvier, Marie-Anne Poursat.—[2nd ed.].
        p. cm. — (Springer series in statistics)
    Rev. ed. of: Statistical tools for nonlinear regression / Sylvie Huet . . . [et al.]. c1996.
    Includes bibliographical references and index.

    1. Regression analysis.   2. Nonlinear theories.   3. Parameter estimation.   I. Bouvier,
Annie.   II. Poursat, Marie-Anne.   III. Statistical tools for nonlinear regression.   IV. Title.
V. Series.
    QA278.2.H84 2003
    519.5′36—dc21

2003050498

ISBN 978-1-4419-2301-1   e-ISBN 978-0-387-21574-7

www.springer-ny.com

Springer-Verlag   New York Berlin Heidelberg
A member of BertelsmannSpringer Science+Business Media GmbH

Contents

Preface to the Second Edition

This second edition contains two additional chapters dealing with binomial, multinomial and Poisson models. If you have to analyze data sets where the response variable is a count or the distribution of individuals in categories, you will be interested in these chapters. Generalized linear models are usually used for modeling these data. They assume that the expected response is linked to a linear predictor through a one-to-one known transformation. We consider extensions of these models by taking into account the cases where such a linearizing transformation does not exist. We call these models generalized nonlinear models. Although they do not fall strictly within the definition of nonlinear regression models, the underlying principles and methods are very similar. In Chapter 6 we consider binomial variables, and in Chapter 7 multinomial and Poisson variables. It is fairly straightforward to extend the method to other distributions such as exponential distribution or gamma distribution.

Maintaining the approach of the first edition, we start by presenting practical examples, and we describe the statistical problems posed by these examples, focusing on those that cannot be analyzed within the framework of generalized linear models. We demonstrate how to solve these problems using **nls2**. It should be noted that we do not review the statistical problems related to generalized linear models that have been discussed extensively in the literature. Rather, we postulate that you have some practical experience with data analysis using generalized linear models, and we base our demonstrations on the link between the generalized nonlinear model and the heteroscedastic nonlinear regression model dealt with in Chapter 3. For that purpose, the estimation method based on the quasi-likelihood equations is introduced in Section 3.3. The use of the **nls2**'s facilities for analyzing data modeled with generalized nonlinear models is the main contribution of the second edition.

The modifications to Chapters 1 to 5 are minor except for the bootstrap method. Indeed, we propose an extension of the bootstrap method to heteroscedastic models in Section 3.4, and we apply it to calculating prediction and calibration confidence intervals.

Let us conclude this preface with the improvements made in **nls2**. The software is now available under Linux and with R^1 as the host system, in addition to the Unix/SPlus version. Moreover, a C/Fortran library, called nls2C, allows the user to carry out estimation without any host system. And, of course, all of the methods discussed in this edition are introduced in the software.

---

[1] http://cran.r-project.org/

Preface to the First Edition

If you need to analyze a data set using a parametric nonlinear regression model, if you are not familiar with statistics and software, and if you make do with S-Plus, this book is for you. In each chapter we start by presenting practical examples. We then describe the statistical problems posed by these examples, and we demonstrate how to solve these problems. Finally, we apply the proposed methods to the example data sets. You will not find any mathematical proofs here. Rather, we try, when possible, to explain the solutions using intuitive arguments. This is really a *cookbook*.

Most of the methods proposed in the book are derived from classical nonlinear regression theory, but we have also made attempts to provide more modern methods that have been proven to perform well in practice. Although the theoretical grounds are not developed here, when appropriate we give some technical background using a sans serif type style. You can skip these passages if you are not interested in this information.

The first chapter introduces several examples from experiments in agronomy and biochemistry, to which we will return throughout the book. Each example illustrates a different problem, and we show how to methodically handle these problems using parametric nonlinear regression models. Because the term *parametric model* means that all of the information in the experiments is assumed to be contained in the parameters occurring in the model, we first demonstrate, in Chapter 1, how to estimate the parameters. In Chapter 2 we describe how to determine the accuracy of the estimators. Chapter 3 introduces some new examples and presents methods for handling nonlinear regression models when the variances are heterogeneous with few or no replications. In Chapter 4 we demonstrate methods for checking if the assumptions on which the statistical analysis is based are accurate, and we provide methods for detecting and correcting any misspecification that might exist. In Chapter 5 we describe how to calculate prediction and calibration confidence intervals.

Because good software is necessary for handling nonlinear regression data, we provide, at the end of each chapter, a step-by-step description of how to treat our examples using **nls2** [BH94], the software we have used throughout this book. **nls2** is a software implemented as an extension of the statistical system S-Plus, available at http://www.inra.fr/bia/J/AB/nls2/, and it offers the capability of implementing all of the methods presented in this book.

Last but not least, we are grateful to Suzie Zweizig for a careful rereading of our English. Thanks to her, we hope that you find this book readable!

Nonlinear Regression Model and Parameter Estimation

In this chapter we describe five examples of experiments in agronomy and bio-chemistry; each illustrates a different problem. Because all of the information in the experiments is assumed to be contained in a set of parameters, we will first describe, in this chapter, the parametric nonlinear regression model and how to estimate the parameters of this model.[1]

1.1 Examples

1.1.1 Pasture Regrowth: Estimating a Growth Curve

In biology, the growth curve is of great interest. In this example (treated by Ratkowsky [Rat83]), we observe the yield of pasture regrowth versus time since the last grazing. The results are reported in Table 1.1 and Figure 1.1. The following model is assumed: The yield at time x_i, Y_i, is written as $Y_i = f(x_i, \theta) + \varepsilon_i$, where $f(x, \theta)$ describes the relationship between the yield and the time x. The errors ε_i are centered random variables ($E(\varepsilon_i) = 0$). Because the measurements are in different experimental units, the errors can be assumed to be independent. Moreover, to complete the regression model, we will assume that the variance of ε_i exists and equals σ^2.

Table 1.1. Data of yield of pasture regrowth versus time (the units are not mentioned)

Time after pasture	9	14	21	28	42	57	63	70	79
Yield	8.93	10.8	18.59	22.33	39.35	56.11	61.73	64.62	67.08

---

[1] We use this sans serif type style when we give technical background. You can skip these passages if you are not interested in this information.

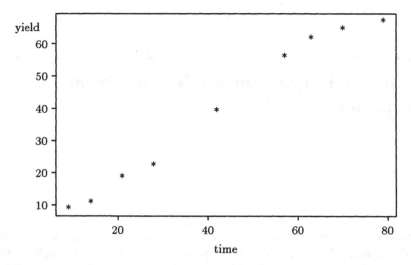

Figure 1.1. Pasture regrowth example: Observed responses versus time

The model under study is the following:

$$\left.\begin{array}{c} Y_i = f(x_i, \theta) + \varepsilon_i \\ \text{Var}(\varepsilon_i) = \sigma^2, \ \text{E}(\varepsilon_i) = 0 \end{array}\right\}.\tag{1.1}$$

In this example, a possible choice for f is the Weibull model:

$$f(x, \theta) = \theta_1 - \theta_2 \exp\left(-\exp(\theta_3 + \theta_4 \log x)\right).\tag{1.2}$$

Depending on the value of θ_4, f presents an inflection point or an exponential increase; see Figure 1.2.

Generally, the choice of the function f depends on knowing the observed biological phenomena. Nevertheless, in this example, Figure 1.1 indicates that the response curve may present an inflection point, making the Weibull model a good choice.

Obviously, it is important to choose the function f well. In this chapter we will show how to estimate the parameters assuming that f is correct. In Chapter 4 we will describe how to validate the choice of f.

1.1.2 Radioimmunological Assay of Cortisol: Estimating a Calibration Curve

Because the amount of hormone contained in a preparation cannot be measured directly, a two-step process is necessary to estimate an unknown dose of hormone. First we must establish *a calibration curve*, and then we invert the calibration curve to find the dose of the hormone.

The calibration curve is estimated by using a radioimmunological assay (or RIA). This assay is based on the fact that the hormone H and its marked

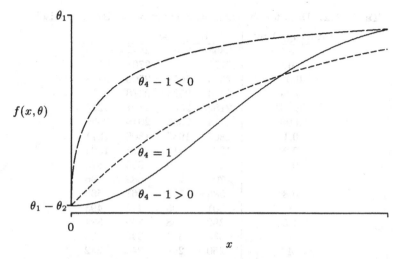

Figure 1.2. Growth models described with the Weibull function defined in Equation (1.2)

isotope H* behave similarly with respect to their specific antibody A. Thus, for fixed quantities of antibody [A] and radioactive hormone [H*], the quantity of linked complex [AH*] decreases when the quantity of cold hormone [H] increases. This property establishes a *calibration curve*. For known dilutions of a purified hormone, the responses [AH*] are measured in terms of c.p.m. (counts per minute). Because the relation between the quantity of linked complex [AH*] and the dose of hormone H varies with the experimental conditions, the calibration curve is evaluated for each assay.

Then, for a preparation containing an unknown quantity of the hormone H, the response [AH*] is measured. The unknown dose is calculated by inverting the calibration curve.

The data for the calibration curve of an RIA of cortisol are given in Table 1.2 (data from the Laboratoire de Physiologie de la Lactation, INRA). Figure 1.3 shows the observed responses as functions of the logarithm of the dose, which is the usual transformation for the x-axis. In this experiment, the response has been observed for the zero dose and the infinite dose. These doses are represented in Figure 1.3 by the values -3 and $+2$, respectively.

The model generally used to describe the variations of the response Y versus the log-dose x is the Richards function (the generalized logistic function). This model depends on five parameters: θ_2, the upper asymptote, is the response for a null dose of hormone H; θ_1, the lower asymptote, is the response for a theoretical infinite dose of H; the other three parameters describe the shape of the decrease of the curve. The equation of the calibration curve is

$$f(x,\theta) = \theta_1 + \frac{\theta_2 - \theta_1}{(1 + \exp(\theta_3 + \theta_4 x))^{\theta_5}}. \qquad (1.3)$$

Table 1.2. Data for the calibration curve of an RIA of cortisol

Dose (ng/.1 ml)	Response (c.p.m.)			
0	2868	2785	2849	2805
0	2779	2588	2701	2752
0.02	2615	2651	2506	2498
0.04	2474	2573	2378	2494
0.06	2152	2307	2101	2216
0.08	2114	2052	2016	2030
0.1	1862	1935	1800	1871
0.2	1364	1412	1377	1304
0.4	910	919	855	875
0.6	702	701	689	696
0.8	586	596	561	562
1	501	495	478	493
1.5	392	358	399	394
2	330	351	343	333
4	250	261	244	242
∞	131	135	134	133

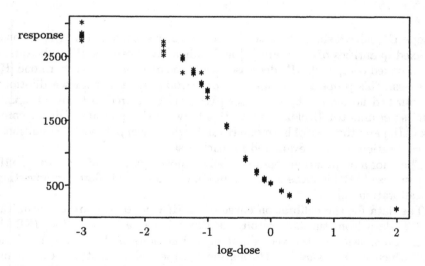

Figure 1.3. Cortisol example: Observed responses (in c.p.m.) versus the logarithms in base 10 of the dose

Once we describe the trend of the variations of Y versus x, we also have to consider the errors $\varepsilon = Y - f(x, \theta)$. Looking carefully at Figure 1.3, we see that the variability of Y depends on the level of the response. For each value of x, with the response Y being observed with replications, the model can be written in the following manner: $Y_{ij} = f(x_i, \theta) + \varepsilon_{ij}$, with j varying from 1 to n_i (n_i equals 8 or 4) and i from 1 to k ($k = 15$). For each value of i the *empirical variance* of the response can be calculated:

$$\left. \begin{array}{l} s_i^2 = \frac{1}{n_i} \sum_{j=1}^{n_i} (Y_{ij} - Y_{i\bullet})^2 \\ \text{with} \quad Y_{i\bullet} = \frac{1}{n_i} \sum_{j=1}^{k} Y_{ij} \end{array} \right\} . \tag{1.4}$$

Table 1.3. Cortisol example: Mean and empirical variance of the response for each value of the dose

Dose	0	0.02	0.04	0.06	0.08
Means: $Y_{i\bullet}$	2765.875	2567.5	2479.75	2194	2053
Variances: s_i^2	6931	4460	4821	5916	1405

Dose	0.1	0.2	0.4	0.6	0.8
Means : $Y_{i\bullet}$	1867	1364.25	889.75	697	576.25
Variances: s_i^2	2288	1518	673	26	230

Dose	1	1.5	2	4	∞
Means: $Y_{i\bullet}$	491.75	385.75	339.25	249.25	133.25
Variances: s_i^2	72	263	69	55	2

Table 1.3 gives the values of s_i^2 and $Y_{i\bullet}$. Because the variance of the response is clearly heterogeneous, it will be assumed that $\text{Var}(\varepsilon_{ij}) = \sigma_i^2$. The model is the following:

$$\left. \begin{array}{l} Y_{ij} = f(x_i, \theta) + \varepsilon_{ij} \\ \text{Var}(\varepsilon_{ij}) = \sigma_i^2, \ \text{E}(\varepsilon_{ij}) = 0 \end{array} \right\} , \tag{1.5}$$

where $j = 1, \ldots n_i$; $i = 1, \ldots k$; and the total number of observations equals $n = \sum_{i=1}^{k} n_i$. f is defined by Equation (1.3), and the ε_{ij} are independent centered random variables. In this experiment, however, we can be even more precise about the heteroscedasticity, that is, about the variations of σ_i^2, because the observations are counts that can safely be assumed to be distributed as Poisson variables, for which variance equals expectation. A reasonable model for the variance could be $\sigma_i^2 = f(x_i, \theta)$, which will be generalized to $\sigma_i^2 = \sigma^2 f(x_i, \theta)^\tau$, where τ can be known or estimated (see Chapter 3).

The aim of this experiment is to estimate an unknown dose of hormone using the calibration curve. Let μ be the expected value of the response for a preparation where the dose of hormone D (or its logarithm X) is unknown; then X is the inverse of f calculated in μ (if μ lies strictly between θ_1 and θ_2):

$$X = f^{-1}(\mu, \theta)$$

$$X = \frac{1}{\theta_4} \left\{ \log \left[\exp \frac{1}{\theta_5} \log \frac{\theta_2 - \theta_1}{\mu - \theta_1} - 1 \right] - \theta_3 \right\}. \tag{1.6}$$

This example will be studied in several places in this book. We will discuss how to estimate the calibration curve and X in this chapter. The problem of calculating the accuracy of the estimation of X will be treated in Chapter 2. Methods for choosing the variance function and testing model specifications will be proposed in Chapter 4. The calibration problem will be treated in detail in Chapter 5. Finally, we show how these data can be fitted using a Poisson nonlinear model in Chapter 7.

1.1.3 Antibodies Anticoronavirus Assayed by an ELISA Test: Comparing Several Response Curves

This experiment uses an ELISA test to detect the presence of anticoronavirus antibodies in the serum of calves and cows. It shows how we can estimate the parameters of two curves together so that we can ultimately determine if the curves are identical up to a horizontal shift. The complete description of the experiment is presented in [HLV87]. Here we limit the problem to the comparison of antibody levels in two serum samples taken in May and June from one cow.

An ELISA test is a collection of observed optical densities, Y, for different serum dilutions, say d. The results are reported in Table 1.4 and Figure 1.4.

Table 1.4. ELISA example: Observed values of Y for the sera taken in May and June. Two values of the response are observed

dilution	Response (Optical Density)			
d	May		June	
1/30	1.909	1.956	1.886	1.880
1/90	1.856	1.876	1.853	1.870
1/270	1.838	1.841	1.747	1.772
1/810	1.579	1.584	1.424	1.406
1/2430	1.057	1.072	0.781	0.759
1/7290	0.566	0.561	0.377	0.376
1/21869	0.225	0.229	0.153	0.138
1/65609	0.072	0.114	0.053	0.058

Assuming that the sera are assayed under the same experimental conditions, the problem is to quantify the differences (in terms of antibody level)

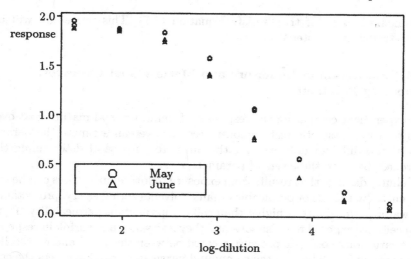

Figure 1.4. ELISA example: Observed responses versus the logarithms of the dilution, $x = -\log_{10} d$

between the sera using their ELISA response curves. For that purpose, the biological assay techniques described in [Fin78] can be used to estimate the *potency* of one serum *relative* to another serum. The potency ρ is defined in the following manner: One unit of serum taken in May is assumed to produce the same response as ρ units of serum taken in June. This means that the two sera must contain the same effective constituent, the antibody, and that all other constituents are without effect on the response. Hence one preparation behaves as a dilution of the other in an inert diluent.

Let $F^{\text{May}}(d)$ and $F^{\text{June}}(d)$ be the response functions for the sera taken in May and June, respectively. If the assumptions defined earlier are fulfilled, then the two regression functions must be related in the following manner: $F^{\text{May}}(d) = F^{\text{June}}(\rho d)$.

The relationship between the optical density Y and the logarithm of the dilution $x = \log_{10}(1/d)$ is usually modeled by a sigmoidal curve: $F^{\text{May}}(d) = f(x, \theta^{\text{May}})$ and $F^{\text{June}}(d) = f(x, \theta^{\text{June}})$, with

$$f(x, \theta) = \theta_1 + \frac{\theta_2 - \theta_1}{1 + \exp \theta_3 (x - \theta_4)}.$$

Thus, the estimation of ρ is based on an assumption of *parallelism* between the two response curves:

$$f(x, \theta^{\text{May}}) = f(x - \beta; \theta^{\text{June}}), \tag{1.7}$$

where $\beta = \log_{10}(1/\rho)$.

In this chapter we will estimate the parameters of the regression functions. Obviously, one must also estimate β. For that purpose, the two curves must be compared to see if they satisfy Equation (1.7). This procedure will be demonstrated in Chapter 2.

1.1.4 Comparison of Immature and Mature Goat Ovocytes: Comparing Parameters

This experiment comparing the responses of immature and mature goat ovocytes to a hyperosmotic test demonstrates how we can estimate the parameters of two different data sets for the ultimate purpose of determining the differences between these sets of parameters.

Cellular damage that results from exposure to low temperatures can be circumvented by the use of permeable organic solvents acting as cryoprotectants. Cell water permeability is higher than cell cryoprotectant permeability. Thus, when cells are exposed to these solvents, they lose water and shrink in response to the variation of osmotic pressure created between the intra- and extracellular compartments. Then, as the compound permeates, water reenters the cell, and the cell reexpands until the system reaches an osmotic equilibrium. The results obtained using immature and ovulated (mature) ovocytes exposed to propane-diol, a permeable compound, are presented in [LGR94].

The cell volume during equilibration is recorded at each time t. In order to obtain water (P_w) and propane-diol (P_S) permeabilities, the following equations are used:

$$\left. \begin{array}{l} \dfrac{V(t)}{V_0} = \dfrac{1}{V_0}(V_w(t) + V_s(t) + V_x), \\[2mm] \dfrac{dV_w}{dt} = P_w\left(\gamma_1 + \gamma_2\dfrac{1}{V_w} + \gamma_3\dfrac{V_s}{V_w}\right) \\[2mm] \dfrac{dV_s}{dt} = P_s\left(\gamma_4 + \gamma_5\dfrac{V_s}{V_w}\right) \end{array} \right\} . \tag{1.8}$$

The first equation expresses the cell volume $V(t)$ as a percentage of initial isotonic cell volume V_0 at any given time t during equilibration; V_x is a known parameter depending on the stage of the oocyte (mature or immature); $V_w(t)$ and $V_s(t)$ are the volumes of intracellular water and cryoprotectant, respectively; and the parameters γ are known. The data are reported in Table 1.5.

In this example, the variations of $Y = V(t)/V_0$ versus the time t are approximated by

$$f(t, P_w, P_s) = \frac{1}{V_0}(V_w(t) + V_s(t) + V_x),$$

where V_w and V_s are the solutions of a system of ordinary differential equations depending on P_w and P_s.

Our aim here is to estimate the parameters P_w and P_s for both types of ovocytes and to compare their values. We also are interested in the temporal evolution of intracellular propane-diol penetration ($V_s(t)$), expressed as the fraction of initial isotonic cell volume V_0.

Table 1.5. Fraction of volume at time t for two stages (mature and immature) of ovocytes

Time	Fraction of Cell Volume for Mature Ovocytes						
0.5	0.6833	0.6870	0.7553	0.6012	0.6655	0.7630	0.7380
1	0.6275	0.5291	0.5837	0.5425	0.5775	0.6640	0.6022
1.5	0.6743	0.5890	0.5837	0.5713	0.6309	0.6960	0.6344
2	0.7290	0.6205	0.5912	0.5936	0.6932	0.7544	0.6849
2.5	0.7479	0.6532	0.6064	0.6164	0.7132	0.7717	0.7200
3	0.7672	0.6870	0.6376	0.6884	0.7494	0.8070	0.7569
4	0.7865	0.7219	0.6456	0.7747	0.8064	0.8342	0.8100
5	0.8265	0.7580	0.6782	0.8205	0.8554	0.8527	0.8424
7	0.8897	0.8346	0.8238	0.8680	0.8955	0.8621	0.8490
10	0.9250	0.9000	0.9622	0.9477	0.9321	0.8809	0.8725
12	0.9480	0.9290	1.0000	0.9700	0.9362	0.8905	0.8930
15	0.9820	0.9550	1.0000	1.0000	0.9784	0.9100	0.9242
20	1.0000	0.9800	1.0000	1.0000	1.0000	0.9592	0.9779
Time	Fraction of Cell Volume for Immature Ovocytes						
0.5	0.4536	0.4690	0.6622	0.621	0.513		
1	0.4297	0.4552	0.5530	0.370	0.425		
1.5	0.4876	0.4690	0.5530	0.400	0.450		
2	0.5336	0.4760	0.5535	0.420	0.475		
2.5	0.5536	0.4830	0.5881	0.460	0.500		
3	0.5618	0.5047	0.6097	0.490	0.550		
3.5	0.6065	0.5269	0.6319	0.520	0.600		
4	0.6365	0.5421	0.6699	0.550	0.650		
4.5	0.6990	0.5814	0.6935	0.570	0.700		
5	0.7533	0.6225	0.7176	0.580	0.750		
6.5	0.7823	0.6655	0.7422	0.630	0.790		
8	0.8477	0.7105	0.7674	0.690	0.830		
10	0.8966	0.8265	0.8464	0.750	0.880		
12	0.9578	0.9105	0.9115	0.800	0.950		
15	1.0000	0.9658	0.9404	0.900	1.000		
20	1.0000	1.0000	0.9800	0.941	1.000		

1.1.5 Isomerization: More than One Independent Variable

These data, given by Carr [Car60] and extensively treated by Bates and Watts [BW88], illustrate how to estimate parameters when there is more than one variable.

The reaction rate of the catalytic isomerization of n-pentane to iso-pentane depends on various factors such as the partial pressures of the needed products (employed to speed up the reaction). The differential reaction rate is expressed as grams of iso-pentane produced per gram of catalyst per hour, and the instantaneous partial pressure of each component is measured. The data are reproduced in Table 1.6.

Table 1.6. Reaction rate of the catalytic isomerization of n-pentane to iso-pentane versus the partial pressures of hydrogen, n-pentane, and iso-pentane

Partial Pressure of			Reaction
Hydrogen	n-Pentane	Iso-Pentane	Rate
205.8	90.9	37.1	3.541
404.8	92.9	36.3	2.397
209.7	174.9	49.4	6.694
401.6	187.2	44.9	4.722
224.9	92.7	116.3	0.593
402.6	102.2	128.9	0.268
212.7	186.9	134.4	2.797
406.2	192.6	134.9	2.451
133.3	140.8	87.6	3.196
470.9	144.2	86.9	2.021
300.0	68.3	81.7	0.896
301.6	214.6	101.7	5.084
297.3	142.2	10.5	5.686
314.0	146.7	157.1	1.193
305.7	142.0	86.0	2.648
300.1	143.7	90.2	3.303
305.4	141.1	87.4	3.054
305.2	141.5	87.0	3.302
300.1	83.0	66.4	1.271
106.6	209.6	33.0	11.648
417.2	83.9	32.9	2.002
251.0	294.4	41.5	9.604
250.3	148.0	14.7	7.754
145.1	291.0	50.2	11.59

A common form of the model is the following:

$$f(x, \theta) = \frac{\theta_1 \theta_3 (P - I/1.632)}{1 + \theta_2 H + \theta_3 P + \theta_4 I}, \qquad (1.9)$$

where x is a three-dimensional variate: $x = (H, P, I)$ where H, P, and I are the partial pressures of hydrogen, n-pentane and iso-pentane, respectively. In this example we will estimate the θ; in Chapter 2 we will calculate the confidence intervals.

1.2 The Parametric Nonlinear Regression Model

We will use the following notation to define the parametric nonlinear regression model: n_i replications of the response Y are observed for each value of the *independent variable* x_i; let Y_{ij}, for $j = 1, \ldots n_i$, be these observations. The total number of observations is $n = \sum_{i=1}^{k} n_i$ and i varies from 1 to k. In

Example 1.1.1, n_i equals 1 for all values of i, and $k = n$. In Example 1.1.5, the variable x is of dimension three: x_i is a vector of values taken by (H, P, I).

It is assumed that the true regression relationship between Y and x is the sum of a systematic part, described by a function $\mu(x)$, and a random part. Generally, the function $\mu(x)$ is unknown and is approximated by a parametric function f, called the *regression function*, that depends on unknown parameters θ:

$$Y_{ij} = f(x_i, \theta) + \varepsilon_{ij}.$$

θ is a vector of p parameters $\theta_1, \theta_2, \ldots \theta_p$. The function f does not need to be known explicitly; in Example 1.1.4, f is a function of the solution of differential equations.

ε is a random *error* equal, by construction, to the discrepancy between Y and $f(x, \theta)$. Let σ_i^2 be the variance of ε_{ij}. The values of σ_i^2, or their variations as functions of x_i, are unknown and must be approximated. In some situations the difference in the variances, $\sigma_i - \sigma_{i+1}$, is small. Thus, there is a high confidence in the approximate homogeneity of the variances, and we can then assume that $\text{Var}(\varepsilon_{ij}) = \sigma^2$. In other cases, because of the nature of the observed response or because of the aspect of the data on a graph, there is evidence against the assumption of *homogeneous errors*. In these cases, the true (unknown) variations of σ_i^2 are approximated by a function g called the variance function such that $\text{Var}(\varepsilon_{ij}) = g(x_i, \sigma^2, \theta, \tau)$. In most cases, g will be assumed to depend on f; for example, $g(x, \sigma^2, \theta, \tau) = \sigma^2 f(x, \theta)^\tau$, where τ is a set of parameters that can be assumed to be known or that have to be estimated.

We simplify the necessary technical assumptions by assuming that each θ_a, $a = 1, \ldots p$, varies in the interior of an interval. The function f is assumed to be twice continuously differentiable with respect to the parameters θ.

1.3 Estimation

Because the problem is to estimate the unknown vector θ, a natural solution is to choose the value of θ that minimizes the distances between the values of $f(x, \theta)$ and the observations of Y. For example, one can choose the value of θ that minimizes the *sum of squares* $C(\theta)$ defined by

$$C(\theta) = \sum_{i=1}^{k} \sum_{j=1}^{n_i} (Y_{ij} - f(x_i, \theta))^2. \tag{1.10}$$

Let $\widehat{\theta}$ be this value. $\widehat{\theta}$ is the *least squares estimator* of θ. If we assume that $\text{Var}(\varepsilon_{ij}) = \sigma^2$, an estimate of σ^2 is obtained as

$$\widehat{\sigma}^2 = \frac{C(\widehat{\theta})}{n}. \tag{1.11}$$

Under the assumptions stated in the preceding paragraph, $\widehat{\theta}$ is also the solution of the set of p equations:

$$\sum_{i=1}^{k} \frac{\partial f}{\partial \theta_a}(x_i, \theta) \sum_{j=1}^{n_i} (Y_{ij} - f(x_i, \theta)) = 0, \tag{1.12}$$

for $a = 1, \ldots p$, where $\partial f / \partial \theta_a$ is the partial derivative of f with respect to θ_a.

Because f is nonlinear in θ, no explicit solution can be calculated. Instead an iterative procedure is needed.

The least squares estimator of θ is also the maximum likelihood estimator in the case of Gaussian observations. Recall the main features of the maximum likelihood method. Let Y be a random variable distributed as a Gaussian variable with expectation $f(x, \theta)$ and variance σ^2. The probability density of Y at point y is defined as follows:

$$\ell(y, x, \theta, \sigma^2) = \frac{1}{\sqrt{2\pi\sigma^2}} \exp\left(-\frac{(y - f(x, \theta))^2}{2\sigma^2}\right).$$

We observe $n = \sum_{i=1}^{k} n_i$ independent Gaussian variables $Y_{ij}, j = 1, \ldots n_i, i = 1, \ldots k$ with expectation $\mathrm{E}(Y_{ij}) = f(x_i, \theta)$ and variance $\mathrm{Var}(Y_{ij}) = \sigma^2$. The probability density of the observations calculated in $y_{ij}, j = 1, \ldots n_i, i = 1, \ldots k$ is equal to the following formula:

$$\prod_{i=1}^{k} \prod_{j=1}^{n_i} \ell(y_{ij}, x_i, \theta, \sigma^2).$$

The *likelihood* is a random variable defined as the probability density calculated in the observations:

$$L(Y_{11}, \ldots, Y_{kn_k}; \theta, \sigma^2) = \prod_{i=1}^{k} \prod_{j=1}^{n_i} \ell(Y_{ij}, x_i, \theta, \sigma^2).$$

The *maximum likelihood estimators* for θ and σ^2 are those values that maximize the likelihood, or equivalently, its logarithm:

$$V(\theta, \sigma^2) = -\frac{n}{2} \log(2\pi\sigma^2) - \frac{1}{2\sigma^2} \sum_{i=1}^{k} \sum_{j=1}^{n_i} (Y_{ij} - f(x_i, \theta))^2.$$

It is clear that maximizing $V(\theta, \sigma^2)$ in θ is equivalent to minimizing $C(\theta)$. The maximum likelihood estimator of σ^2 will satisfy that the derivative of $V(\theta, \sigma^2)$ with respect to σ^2 equals 0. Namely, we get the following:

$$\frac{\partial V}{\partial \sigma^2} = -\frac{n}{2\sigma^2} + \frac{1}{2\sigma^4} C(\theta) = 0$$

leads to Equation (1.11).

In the case of *heterogeneous variances* ($\mathrm{Var}(\varepsilon_{ij}) = \sigma_i^2$), it is natural to favor observations with small variances by weighting the sum of squares. The σ_i^2 are unknown, so they must be replaced by an estimate. If each n_i is big enough, say 4, as in Example 1.1.2, then σ_i^2 can be estimated by s_i^2, the empirical variance (see Equation (1.4)). The *weighted sum of squares* is

$$W(\theta) = \sum_{i=1}^{k} \sum_{j=1}^{n_i} \frac{(Y_{ij} - f(x_i, \theta))^2}{s_i^2}, \qquad (1.13)$$

and the value of θ that minimizes $W(\theta)$ is the *weighted least squares estimator* of θ. The problem of estimating the parameters in heteroscedastic models is treated more generally in Chapter 3.

1.4 Applications

1.4.1 Pasture Regrowth: Parameter Estimation and Graph of Observed and Adjusted Response Values

Model The regression function is

$$f(x, \theta) = \theta_1 - \theta_2 \exp\left(-\exp(\theta_3 + \theta_4 \log x)\right),$$

and the variances are homogeneous: $\text{Var}(\varepsilon_i) = \sigma^2$.

Method The parameters are estimated by minimizing the sum of squares $C(\theta)$; see Equation (1.10).

Results

Parameters	Estimated Values
θ_1	69.95
θ_2	61.68
θ_3	−9.209
θ_4	2.378

The *adjusted response curve*, $f(x, \widehat{\theta})$, is shown in Figure 1.5. It is defined by the following equation:

$$f(x, \widehat{\theta}) = 69.95 - 61.68 \exp\left(-\exp(-9.209 + 2.378 \log x)\right).$$

1.4.2 Cortisol Assay: Parameter Estimation and Graph of Observed and Adjusted Response Values

Model The regression function is

$$f(x, \theta) = \theta_1 + \frac{\theta_2 - \theta_1}{(1 + \exp(\theta_3 + \theta_4 x))^{\theta_5}},$$

and the variances are heterogeneous: $\text{Var}(\varepsilon_i) = \sigma_i^2$.

Method The parameters are estimated by minimizing the weighted sum of squares $W(\theta)$; see Equation (1.13).

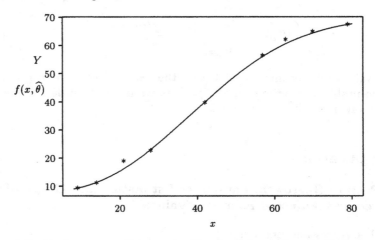

Figure 1.5. Pasture regrowth example: Graph of observed and adjusted response values

Results

Parameters	Estimated Values
θ_1	133.30
θ_2	2759.8
θ_3	3.0057
θ_4	3.1497
θ_5	0.64309

The adjusted response curve, $f(x, \widehat{\theta})$, is shown in Figure 1.6. It is defined by the following equation:

$$f(x, \widehat{\theta}) = 133.3 + \frac{2759.8 - 133.3}{(1 + \exp(3.0057 + 3.1497x))^{0.64309}}.$$

1.4.3 ELISA Test: Parameter Estimation and Graph of Observed and Adjusted Curves for May and June

Model The regression function is

$$f(x, \theta) = \theta_1 + \frac{\theta_2 - \theta_1}{1 + \exp \theta_3 (x - \theta_4)},$$

and the variances are homogeneous: $\text{Var}(\varepsilon_i) = \sigma^2$.

Method The parameters are estimated by minimizing the sum of squares $C(\theta)$; see Equation (1.10).

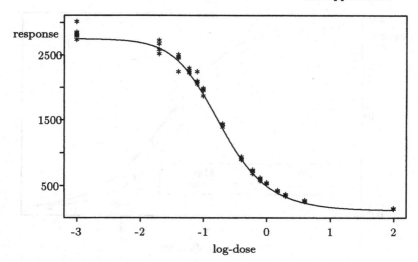

Figure 1.6. Cortisol assay example: Graph of observed and adjusted response values

Results

Parameters	Estimated Values
θ_1^{May}	0.04279
θ_2^{May}	1.936
θ_3^{May}	2.568
θ_4^{May}	3.467
θ_1^{June}	0.0581
θ_2^{June}	1.909
θ_3^{June}	2.836
θ_4^{June}	3.251

The adjusted response curves for May and June are shown in Figure 1.7.

1.4.4 Ovocytes: Parameter Estimation and Graph of Observed and Adjusted Volume of Mature and Immature Ovocytes in Propane-Diol

Model The regression function is

$$f(t, P_w, P_s) = \frac{1}{V_0}(V_w(t) + V_s(t) + V_x),$$

where V_w and V_s are solutions of Equation (1.8). The variances are homogeneous: $\text{Var}(\varepsilon_i) = \sigma^2$.

Method The parameters are estimated by minimizing the sum of squares $C(\theta)$; see Equation (1.10).

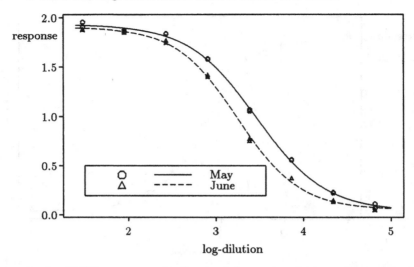

Figure 1.7. ELISA test example: Graph of observed and adjusted curves for May and June

Results

	Parameters	Estimated Values
Mature	P_w	0.0784
ovocytes	P_s	0.00147
Immature	P_w	0.1093
ovocytes	P_s	0.00097

The adjusted response curves for mature and immature ovocytes are shown in Figure 1.8.

1.4.5 Isomerization: Parameter Estimation and Graph of Adjusted versus Observed Values

Model The regression function is

$$f(x, \theta) = \frac{\theta_1 \theta_3 (P - I/1.632)}{1 + \theta_2 H + \theta_3 P + \theta_4 I},$$

where x is a three-dimensional variate, $x = (H, P, I)$, and where the variances are homogeneous: $\text{Var}(\varepsilon_i) = \sigma^2$.

Method The parameters are estimated by minimizing the sum of squares $C(\theta)$; see Equation (1.10).

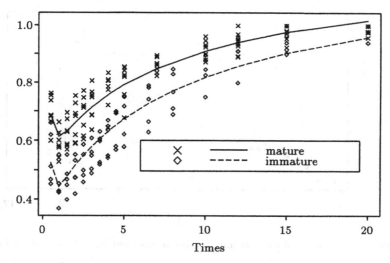

Figure 1.8. Ovocytes example: Graph of observed and adjusted volume of mature and immature ovocytes in propane-diol

Results

Parameters	Estimated Values
θ_1	35.9191
θ_2	0.07086
θ_3	0.03774
θ_4	0.1672

Figure 1.9 shows the values of the adjusted response curve, $f(x_i, \widehat{\theta})$, versus the observations Y_i. $f(x, \widehat{\theta})$ is defined by the following equation:

$$f(x, \widehat{\theta}) = \frac{1.356(P - I/1.632)}{1 + 0.071H + 0.038P + 0.167I}.$$

1.5 Conclusion and References

For each example presented here, we chose a model for the response curve and calculated an estimate of the parameters, but we still need to assess the accuracy of our estimates. Consider the RIA example: We were able to calculate an estimate of X, the inverse of f calculated in a known value μ; however, now we need to calculate the accuracy of this estimate. For the ELISA data, we estimated two response curves, but we are interested in testing the hypothesis of parallelism between these curves. In Example 1.1.4, we wanted to calculate confidence regions for the pair (P_w, P_s).

The next chapter describes the tools that help us answer these questions.

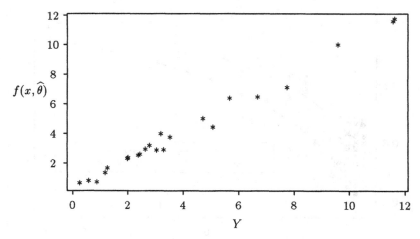

Figure 1.9. Isomerization example: Graph of adjusted versus observed values

For more information, the interested reader can find a complete description of statistical and numerical methods in nonlinear regression models in the book of G. Seber and C. Wild [SW89]. See also the book of H. Bunke and O. Bunke [BB89] and the book of A. Gallant [Gal87]. These are strong in theory and cover mainly the case of homogeneous variances. Users of econometrics should be interested in the third one, which covers the field of multivariate nonlinear regressions and dynamic nonlinear models. The books of S. Huet et al. [HJM91] and R. Carroll and D. Ruppert [CR88] consider the case of heterogeneous variances. Response curves that are currently used in biological frameworks are described in the books of D. Ratkowsky [Rat89], J. Lebreton and C. Millier [LM82]. Other books are concerned with specific subjects, such as the books of D. Bates and D. Watts [BW88] and D. Ratkowsky [Rat83] about nonlinear curvatures, the book of G. Ross [Ros90] about parameter transformations, and the book of V. Fedorov and P. Hackl [FH97] about optimal designs. The book of W. Venables and B. Ripley [VR94] shows how to analyze data using S-Plus.

1.6 Using nls2

This section reproduces the commands and files used in this chapter to treat the examples by using **nls2**. We assume that the user is familiar with S-Plus and has access to the help files of **nls2**, which provide all of the necessary information about syntax and possibilities.

The outputs are not reproduced; the main results are shown in the preceding part.

Typographical Conventions We use the prompt **$** for the operating system commands and the prompt **>** for the S-Plus commands. Continuation lines are indented.

Pasture Regrowth Example

Creating the Data

The experimental data (Table 1.1, page 1) are stored in a *dataframe* structure:

```
$ Splus
> pasture <- data.frame(
    time=c(9, 14, 21, 28, 42, 57, 63, 70, 79),
    yield= c(8.93, 10.8, 18.59, 22.33, 39.35,
            56.11, 61.73, 64.62, 67.08))
```

Plot of the Observed Yield versus Time

We plot the observed values of yield versus time using the function **pldnls2**:

```
> library("nls2") # attach the nls2 library
> X11()           # open a graphical device
> pldnls2(pasture, response.name="yield", X.name="time",
          title = "Pasture regrowth example",
          sub = "Observed response")
```

(See Figure 1.1, page 2.)

Description of the Model

The model defined in Section 1.4.1, page 13, is described using a symbolic syntax in a file called **pasture.mod1**:

```
resp yield;
varind time;
parresp p1, p2, p3, p4;
subroutine;
begin
yield=p1-p2*exp(-exp(p3+p4*log(time)));
end
```

Parameter Estimation

Parameters are estimated using the function **nls2**.

Before calling **nls2**, it is necessary to load the programs of the system **nls2** into the S-Plus session; this is done with the function **loadnls2**.

The arguments of **nls2** are the name of the *dataframe*, the name of the file that describes the model, and information about the statistical context, which includes the starting values of the parameters and possibly some other things, as the user chooses. Here we include, for example, the maximum number of iterations:

```
> loadnls2() # load the programs
> pasture.nl1 <- nls2(pasture, "pasture.mod1",
               list(theta.start= c(70, 60, 0, 1), max.iters=100))
>    # Print the estimated values of the parameters
> cat( "Estimated values of the parameters:\n ")
> print( pasture.nl1$theta); cat( "\n\n")
```

(Results are given in Section 1.4.1, page 13.)

Plot of the Observed and Fitted Yields versus Time

We plot the observed and fitted response values versus time using the function plfit:

```
> plfit(pasture.nl1, title = "Pasture regrowth example",
        sub = "Observed and fitted response")
```

(See Figure 1.5, page 14.)

Cortisol Assay Example

Creating the Data

The experimental data (see Table 1.2, page 4) are stored in a *dataframe*. We set the value of the zero dose to 0 and the value of the infinity dose to 10:

```
> corti <- data.frame(dose=c(
    rep(0,8),    rep(0.02,4), rep(0.04,4), rep(0.06,4),
    rep(0.08,4),rep(0.1,4),   rep(0.2,4),   rep(0.4,4),
    rep(0.6,4),  rep(0.8,4),   rep(1,4),     rep(1.5,4),
    rep(2,4),    rep(4,4),     rep(10,4)),
                    cpm=c(
    2868,2785,2849,2805,2779,2588,2701,2752,
    2615,2651,2506,2498,2474,2573,2378,2494,
    2152,2307,2101,2216,2114,2052,2016,2030,
    1862,1935,1800,1871,1364,1412,1377,1304,
    910,919,855,875,702,701,689,696,
    586,596,561,562,501,495,478,493,
    392,358,399,394,330,351,343,333,
    250,261,244,242,131,135,134, 133))
```

Plot of the Observed Responses versus the Logarithm of the Dose

We plot the observed responses versus the logarithm of the dose using the graphical function plot of S-Plus:

```
> logdose<-c(rep(-3,8),log10(corti$dose[9:60]),rep(2,4))
> plot(logdose,corti$cpm,xlab="log-dose",ylab="response",
       title="Cortisol example",sub="Observed cpm")
```

(See Figure 1.3, page 4.)

Description of the Model

The model, defined in Section 1.4.2, page 13, is described in a file called
corti.mod1.

The parameters `minf` and `pinf`, introduced by the key word `pbisresp`,
are the minimal and maximal values accepted for the dose. They do not need
to be estimated; they will be called *second-level parameters*:

```
resp cpm;
varind dose;
parresp n,d,a,b,g;
pbisresp minf,pinf;
subroutine;
begin
cpm= if dose <= minf then d else
        if dose >= pinf then n else
        n+(d-n)*exp(-g*log(1+exp(a+b*log10(dose))))
     fi fi;
end
```

Parameter Estimation

The function **nls2** is used to estimate the parameters. Its first argument is
the name of the *dataframe*, its second argument describes the model, and its
third contains the starting values of the parameters.

The second argument, which describes the model, includes the name of
the description file, the values of the *second-level parameters*, and information
about the variance (VI means "variance intrareplications"):

```
> corti.nl1<-nls2(corti,
    list(file="corti.mod1", gamf=c(0,10),vari.type="VI"),
    c(3000,30,0,1,1))
>   # Print the estimated values of the parameters
> cat( "Estimated values of the parameters:\n ")
> print( corti.nl1$theta); cat( "\n\n")
```

(Results are given in Section 1.4.2, page 13.)

Plot of the oObserved and Fitted Response Values

We plot the observed and fitted response values versus the logarithm of the
dose by using graphical functions of S-Plus:

```
> plot(logdose,corti$cpm,xlab="log-dose",ylab="response",
        title="Cortisol example",sub="Observed and fitted response")
> lines(unique(logdose),corti.nl1$response)
```

(See Figure 1.6, page 15.)

ELISA Test Example

Creating the Data

The experimental data (see Table 1.4, page 6) are stored in a *dataframe*. The independent variable is equal to $\log_{10}$ of the dilution. The curves are called m for May and j for June:

```
> dilution <-rep(c(
      rep(30,2), rep(90,2), rep(270,2), rep(810,2),
      rep(2430,2), rep(7290,2), rep(21869,2), rep(65609,2)), 2)
> elisa <- data.frame(logd=log10(dilution),
          OD=c(1.909, 1.956, 1.856, 1.876, 1.838, 1.841, 1.579,
               1.584, 1.057, 1.072, 0.566, 0.561, 0.225, 0.229,
               0.072, 0.114, 1.886, 1.880, 1.853, 1.870, 1.747,
               1.772, 1.424, 1.406, 0.781, 0.759, 0.377, 0.376,
               0.153, 0.138, 0.053, 0.058),
          curves=c(rep("m", 16), rep("j", 16))))
```

Plot of the Observed Responses versus the Logarithm of the Dilution

We plot the observed response values versus the logarithm of the dilution using the function pldnls2:

```
> pldnls2(elisa,response.name="OD",X.names="logd")
```

(See Figure 1.4, page 7.)

Description of the Model

The model defined in Section 1.4.3, page 14, is described in a file called elisa.mod1:

```
resp OD;
varind logd;
aux a1;
parresp p1,p2,p3,p4;
subroutine;
begin
a1= 1+exp(p3*(logd-p4));
OD=p1+(p2-p1)/a1;
end
```

Parameter Estimation

To estimate the parameters, we use the function nls2:

```
> elisa.nl1<-nls2(elisa,"elisa.mod1",rep(c(2,0,1,0),2))
> cat( "Estimated values of the parameters:\n ")
> print( elisa.nl1$theta); cat( "\n\n")
```

(Results are given in Section 1.4.3, page 14.)

Plot of the Observed and Fitted Curves

We plot the observed and fitted response values using the function `plfit`:

```
> plfit(elisa.nl1, title="ELISA assay")
```

(See Figure 1.7, page 16.)

Ovocytes Example

Creating the Data

The *dataframe* is created from the values of the time and the volumes of ovocytes. The two curves are called m for mature ovocytes and i for immature ovocytes (see Table 1.5, page 9):

```
> Times <- c( rep(0.5,7),rep(1,7),rep(1.5,7),rep(2,7),
        rep(2.5,7),rep(3,7),rep(4,7),rep(5,7),
        rep(7,7),rep(10,7),rep(12,7),rep(15,7),rep(20,7),
        rep(0.5,5),rep(1,5),rep(1.5,5),rep(2,5),
        rep(2.5,5),rep(3,5),rep(3.5,5), rep(4,5), rep(4.5,5),
        rep(5,5), rep(6.5,5),rep(8,5), rep(10,5),rep(12,5),
        rep(15,5),rep(20,5))
> V <- c (0.6833, 0.6870, 0.7553, 0.6012, 0.6655, 0.7630, 0.7380,
        0.6275, 0.5291, 0.5837, 0.5425, 0.5775, 0.6640, 0.6022,
        0.6743, 0.5890, 0.5837, 0.5713, 0.6309, 0.6960, 0.6344,
        0.7290, 0.6205, 0.5912, 0.5936, 0.6932, 0.7544, 0.6849,
        0.7479, 0.6532, 0.6064, 0.6164, 0.7132, 0.7717, 0.7200,
        0.7672, 0.6870, 0.6376, 0.6884, 0.7494, 0.8070, 0.7569,
        0.7865, 0.7219, 0.6456, 0.7747, 0.8064, 0.8342, 0.8100,
        0.8265, 0.7580, 0.6782, 0.8205, 0.8554, 0.8527, 0.8424,
        0.8897, 0.8346, 0.8238, 0.8680, 0.8955, 0.8621, 0.8490,
        0.9250, 0.9000, 0.9622, 0.9477, 0.9321, 0.8809, 0.8725,
        0.9480, 0.9290, 1.0000, 0.9700, 0.9362, 0.8905, 0.8930,
        0.9820, 0.9550, 1.0000, 1.0000, 0.9784, 0.9100, 0.9242,
        1.0000, 0.9800, 1.0000, 1.0000, 1.0000, 0.9592, 0.9779,
        0.4536, 0.4690, 0.6622, 0.6210, 0.5130,
        0.4297, 0.4552, 0.5530, 0.3700, 0.4250,
        0.4876, 0.4690, 0.5530, 0.4000, 0.4500,
        0.5336, 0.4760, 0.5535, 0.4200, 0.4750,
        0.5536, 0.4830, 0.5881, 0.4600, 0.5000,
        0.5618, 0.5047, 0.6097, 0.4900, 0.5500,
        0.6065, 0.5269, 0.6319, 0.5200, 0.6000,
        0.6365, 0.5421, 0.6699, 0.5500, 0.6500,
        0.6990, 0.5814, 0.6935, 0.5700, 0.7000,
        0.7533, 0.6225, 0.7176, 0.5800, 0.7500,
        0.7823, 0.6655, 0.7422, 0.6300, 0.7900,
        0.8477, 0.7105, 0.7674, 0.6900, 0.8300,
        0.8966, 0.8265, 0.8464, 0.7500, 0.8800,
```

```
            0.9578, 0.9105, 0.9115, 0.8000, 0.9500,
            1.0000, 0.9658, 0.9404, 0.9000, 1.0000,
            1.0000, 1.0000, 0.9800, 0.9410, 1.0000)
> ovo <- data.frame(T=Times,V, curves=c(rep("m", 91), rep("i", 80)))
```

Description of the Model

The model defined in Section 1.4.4, page 15, is described in a file called
ovo.mod1. The known parameters are declared to be *second-level parameters*, except for the parameter called ov, whose value depends on the curve.
The value of ov will be set by numerical equality constraints when calling
nls2:

```
resp V;
varind T;
parresp Pw, Ps, ov;
varint t;
valint T;
pbisresp mm, mv, mo, mme, mve, Vo, a, moe, moi, phi;
aux z1, z3, g1,g2,g3,g4,g5;
F Vw, Vs;
dF dVw, dVs;
subroutine;
begin
z1 = Vo*(1-ov)*moi/1e+3;
z3 = a*phi*mv/mm ;
g1 = -a*(mme/mve)*(moe+mo)/1e+3;
g2 = (mme/mve)*a*z1;
g3 = (mme/mve)*z3;
g4 = (mm/mv)*a*mo/1e+3;
g5 = -a*phi;
dVw = Pw*(g1 + g2/Vw + g3*Vs/Vw);
dVs = Ps*(g4 + g5*Vs/Vw);
V = Vw[T]/Vo + Vs[T]/Vo + ov;
end
```

A C Program to Calculate the Model

The system **nls2** includes the possibility of generating a C Program from
the formal description of the model. Once compiled and loaded into the S-
Plus session, this program is used by the function **nls2** instead of the default
evaluation, that is, evaluation by syntaxical trees. Using C programs reduces
execution time and saves memory space. Here, because the model is especially
complicated, we use this option.

The operating system command **analDer**, provided with the system **nls2**,
generates a C routine in a file called ovo.mod1.c:

```
$  analDer ovo.mod1
```

The file is loaded into the S-Plus session using the function loadnls2:

```
> loadnls2("ovo.mod1.c")
```

Parameter Estimation

To estimate the parameters, the function nls2 is called with four arguments: the name of the *dataframe*, a list that describes the model, ovo.mod1, the starting values of the parameters, and a list that gives information about the ordinary differential equation system, ovo.int.

ovo.mod1 includes the name of the description file, the values of the *second-level parameters*, and a component called eq.theta, which contains the values of the numerical equality constraints on the parameters. With these constraints, we set the parameter ov to its known value. The value NaN (NotANumber) means that no constraint is set on the corresponding parameter.

ovo.int includes the initial value of the integration variable, the number of parameters in the system, and its initial values (a matrix with two rows, one for each curve, and two columns, one for each equation of the system):

```
> ovo.mod1<-  # The list that describes the model
      list(file="ovo.mod1",
      gamf=c(76.09, 1.04, 1.62, 18,1,1.596e-6,6.604e-4,0.29,0.29,1),
      eq.theta=c(NaN, NaN,   0.15,   NaN, NaN,   0.065))
> ovo.int<-   # The list that describes the integration context
      list(start=0, nb.theta.odes=3,
      cond.start=matrix(c(1.35660e-6, 0, 1.49226e-06, 0), ncol=2))
> ovo.nl1<-nls2(ovo,
                ovo.mod1,
                c(0.1, 0.01,   0.15, 0.1, 0.01, 0.065),
                integ.ctx=ovo.int)
> cat( "Estimated values of the parameters:\n ")
> print( ovo.nl1$theta); cat( "\n\n")
```

(Results are given in Section 1.4.4, page 15.)

Plot of the Results

We plot the observed and fitted response values using function plfit:

```
> plfit(ovo.nl1, title="Ovocytes example")
```

(See Figure 1.8, page 17.)

Isomerization Example

Creating the Data

The *dataframe* includes three independent variables: H for hydrogen, P for n-pentane, and I for iso-pentane. The response values are the observed rates, r (see Table 1.6, page 10):

```
> isomer <- data.frame(
  H=c(205.8, 404.8, 209.7, 401.6, 224.9, 402.6, 212.7,
      406.2, 133.3, 470.9, 300.0, 301.6, 297.3, 314.0,
      305.7, 300.1, 305.4, 305.2, 300.1, 106.6, 417.2,
      251.0, 250.3, 145.1),
  P=c(90.9, 92.9, 174.9, 187.2, 92.7, 102.2, 186.9, 192.6,
      140.8, 144.2, 68.3, 214.6, 142.2, 146.7, 142.0, 143.7,
      141.1, 141.5, 83.0, 209.6, 83.9, 294.4, 148.0, 291.0),
  I=c(37.1, 36.3, 49.4, 44.9, 116.3, 128.9, 134.4, 134.9,
      87.6, 86.9, 81.7, 101.7, 10.5, 157.1, 86.0, 90.2, 87.4,
      87.0, 66.4, 33.0, 32.9, 41.5, 14.7, 50.2),
  r=c(3.541, 2.397, 6.694, 4.722, 0.593, 0.268, 2.797, 2.451,
      3.196, 2.021, 0.896, 5.084, 5.686, 1.193, 2.648, 3.303,
      3.054, 3.302, 1.271, 11.648, 2.002, 9.604, 7.754, 11.590))
```

Description of the Model

The model defined in Section 1.4.5, page 16, is described in a file called
isomer.mod1:

```
resp r;
varind H,P,I;
aux a1, a2;
parresp t1,t2,t3,t4;
subroutine;
begin
a1= t1*t3*(P-I/1.632);
a2= 1+t2*H+t3*P+t4*I;
r=a1/a2;
end
```

Parameter Estimation

To estimate the parameters, the function nls2 is called. Its arguments are
the name of the *dataframe*, the name of the file that describes the model, and
a list of information about the statistical context: the starting values of the
parameters and the requested maximal number of iterations:

```
> loadnls2() # load the programs
> isomer.nl1<-nls2(isomer,"isomer.mod1",
      list(theta.start=c(10,1,1,1), max.iters=100))
> cat( "Estimated values of the parameters:\n ")
> print( isomer.nl1$theta); cat( "\n\n")
```

(Results are given in Section 1.4.5, page 16.)

Plot of the Fitted Values versus the Observed Values

We plot the fitted values versus the observed values using the function plfit:

```
> plfit(isomer.nl1, wanted=list(O.F=T),
        title="Isomerization example")
```

(See Figure 1.9, page 18.)

2

Accuracy of Estimators, Confidence Intervals and Tests

To determine the accuracy of the estimates that we made in Chapter 1, we demonstrate how to calculate confidence intervals and perform tests. The specific concerns of each particular experiment are described herein. We then introduce the methodology, first describing classical asymptotic procedures and two asymptotic tests, the Wald test and the likelihood ratio test, and then we present procedures and tests based on a resampling method, the bootstrap. As before, we conclude the chapter by applying these methods to the examples.

2.1 Examples

Let us assume that in Example 1.1.1 we are interested in the maximum yield, θ_1. We have calculated one estimate of θ_1, $\widehat{\theta}_1 = 69.95$; however, if we do another experiment under the same experimental conditions, the observed values of Y and the estimates of the parameters will be different. Thus, knowing one estimate is not entirely satisfactory; we need to quantify its accuracy.

In Example 1.1.2, we calculated an estimate of the calibration curve. Suppose we now want to estimate the dose of hormone D contained in a preparation that has the expected response $\mu = 2000$ c.p.m. To do this, we must use Equation (1.6), replacing the parameters with their estimates. We find $\widehat{X} = -1.1033$ and $\widehat{D} = \exp \widehat{X} \log 10 = 0.3318$ ng/.1 ml, but we now need to calculate how much confidence we can place in this estimate.

Let us consider Example 1.1.3, in which we estimated two ELISA response curves. Our concern in this experiment was to estimate the relative potency of the two different sera. In order to do this, however, we must verify whether the condition of *parallelism*, as expressed in Equation (1.7), is true. If it does exist for all values of x, then the parameters satisfy that $\theta_1^{\text{May}} = \theta_1^{\text{June}}$, $\theta_2^{\text{May}} = \theta_2^{\text{June}}$, $\theta_3^{\text{May}} = \theta_3^{\text{June}}$. In this case, $\beta = \theta_4^{\text{May}} - \theta_4^{\text{June}}$ is the horizontal distance between the two curves at the inflection point. To determine parallelism we will first test whether these relations between the parameters are true or, more exactly, if they do not contradict the data. If the test does not reject the hypothesis of parallelism, we will be able to estimate β and test if it is significantly different from zero.

In Example 1.1.4 we were interested in comparing parameters P_w and P_s. Because water permeability in cells is higher than propane-diol permeability, water flows out of the cells more rapidly than the propane-diol flows in, resulting in high cell shrinkage. Thus we are interested in the speed of intracellular propane-diol penetration; the cryoprotectant must permeate the ovocytes in a short time. To this end, we will compare the values of V_s at times $T_1 = 1$ mn, $T_2 = 5$ mn, and so on.

Using Example 1.1.5, we will compare different methods for calculating confidence intervals for the parameters.

In sum, what we want to do in all of these examples is to determine if we estimated the function of the parameters denoted $\lambda(\theta)$ accurately. In the first example, $\lambda = \theta_1$, and in the second example, $\lambda = \exp(X \log 10)$, where X is defined by

$$X = \frac{1}{\theta_4} \left\{ \log \left[\exp \frac{1}{\theta_5} \log \frac{\theta_2 - \theta_1}{\mu - \theta_1} - 1 \right] - \theta_3 \right\}.$$

In the third example, if the hypothesis of parallelism is not rejected, we are interested in $\lambda = \beta$ or $\lambda = \exp -\beta$. In the fourth example we are interested in the pairs (P_w, P_s) for each curve, in $\lambda = V_s(T_1)$, and, in $\lambda = V_s(T_2)$.

2.2 Problem Formulation

The nonlinear regression model was defined in Section 1.2. Let $\widehat{\theta}$ be the least squares estimator of θ when we have homogeneous variances, and let it be the weighted least squares estimator of θ when we have heterogeneous[1] variances (see Section 1.3).

Let λ be a function of the parameters and $\widehat{\lambda}$ an estimator of λ: $\widehat{\lambda} = \lambda(\widehat{\theta})$. In this chapter, we will describe how to calculate a confidence interval for λ, and how to do a test.

The function λ must satisfy some *regularity* assumptions. It must be a continuous function of θ with continuous partial derivatives with respect to θ.

2.3 Solutions

2.3.1 Classical Asymptotic Results

$\widehat{\theta}$ is a function of the Y_{ij}, and when the number of observations tends to infinity, its distribution is known: $\widehat{\theta} - \theta$ tends to 0, and the *limiting distribution*

---

[1] See Chapter 3 for a complete treatment when the variance of errors is not constant.

of $V_{\widehat{\theta}}^{-1/2}(\widehat{\theta} - \theta)$ is a standard p-dimensional normal (Gaussian) distribution $\mathcal{N}(0, \mathbf{I}_p)$ with expectation 0 and variance $\mathbf{I}_p$, where $\mathbf{I}_p$ is the $p \times p$ identity matrix and $V_{\widehat{\theta}}$ is the estimated asymptotic *covariance matrix* of $\widehat{\theta}$. Thus, for sufficiently large n, the distribution of $\widehat{\theta}$ may be approximated by the normal distribution $\mathcal{N}(\theta, V_{\widehat{\theta}})$.

We need a result for $\widehat{\lambda} = \lambda(\widehat{\theta})$. The limiting distribution (when n tends to infinity) of

$$\widehat{T} = \frac{\widehat{\lambda} - \lambda}{\widehat{S}}$$

will be a centered normal distribution, $\mathcal{N}(0, 1)$, where $\widehat{S}$ is an estimate of the standard error of $\widehat{\lambda}$.

Notations and Formulas: f_i is for $f(x_i, \theta)$. The p vector of derivatives of f with respect to θ calculated in x_i is denoted by $\partial f_i / \partial \theta$. The components of $\partial f_i / \partial \theta$ are $[(\partial f / \partial \theta_a)(x_i, \theta)]$, $a = 1, \ldots p$.

Let Γ_θ be the $p \times p$ matrix defined as follows:

$$\Gamma_\theta = \frac{1}{\sigma^2} \frac{1}{n} \sum_{i=1}^{k} n_i \frac{\partial f_i}{\partial \theta} \left(\frac{\partial f_i}{\partial \theta}\right)^T,$$

where the exponent T means that the vector is transposed. The elements (a, b) of Γ_θ are

$$\Gamma_{\theta, ab} = \frac{1}{\sigma^2} \frac{1}{n} \sum_{i=1}^{k} n_i \frac{\partial f_i}{\partial \theta_a} \frac{\partial f_i}{\partial \theta_b}.$$

Let Δ_θ be the $p \times p$ matrix

$$\frac{1}{n} \sum_{i=1}^{k} \frac{n_i}{\sigma_i^2} \frac{\partial f_i}{\partial \theta} \left(\frac{\partial f_i}{\partial \theta}\right)^T.$$

Let $\widehat{f}_i = f(x_i, \widehat{\theta})$, $\partial \widehat{f}_i / \partial \theta$ be the vector with components $\partial f / \partial \theta_a(x_i, \widehat{\theta})$, and $\Gamma_{\widehat{\theta}}$ and $\Delta_{\widehat{\theta}}$ be the matrices Γ_θ and Δ_θ, where the unknown parameters are replaced by their estimators:

$$\Gamma_{\widehat{\theta}} = \frac{1}{\widehat{\sigma}^2} \frac{1}{n} \sum_{i=1}^{k} n_i \frac{\partial \widehat{f}_i}{\partial \theta} \left(\frac{\partial \widehat{f}_i}{\partial \theta}\right)^T, \quad \Delta_{\widehat{\theta}} = \frac{1}{n} \sum_{i=1}^{k} \frac{n_i}{\widehat{\sigma}_i^2} \frac{\partial \widehat{f}_i}{\partial \theta} \left(\frac{\partial \widehat{f}_i}{\partial \theta}\right)^T,$$

and $\widehat{\sigma}^2 = C(\widehat{\theta})/n$, $\widehat{\sigma}_i^2 = s_i^2$.

$V_{\widehat{\theta}}$ is the estimate of V_θ, the $p \times p$ asymptotic covariance matrix of $\widehat{\theta}$:

In the case $\mathrm{Var}(\varepsilon_{ij}) = \sigma^2$, $V_{\widehat{\theta}} = \frac{1}{n} \Gamma_{\widehat{\theta}}^{-1}$,

In the case $\mathrm{Var}(\varepsilon_{ij}) = \sigma_i^2$, $V_{\widehat{\theta}} = \frac{1}{n} \Delta_{\widehat{\theta}}^{-1}$.

Because $\widehat{\theta} - \theta$ is small, we get the limiting distribution of $\widehat{\lambda}$ by approximating $\lambda(\widehat{\theta}) - \lambda(\theta)$ by a linear function of $\widehat{\theta} - \theta$:

$$\left(\frac{\partial \lambda}{\partial \theta}\right)^T (\widehat{\theta} - \theta) = \sum_{a=1}^p \frac{\partial \lambda}{\partial \theta_a}(\widehat{\theta}_a - \theta_a).$$

Thus $(\widehat{\lambda} - \lambda)/S_{\widehat{\theta}}$ is distributed, when n tends to infinity, as an $\mathcal{N}(0,1)$ (a Gaussian centered variate with variance 1), where

$$S_\theta^2 = \left(\frac{\partial \lambda}{\partial \theta}\right)^T V_\theta \frac{\partial \lambda}{\partial \theta} = \sum_{a=1}^p \sum_{b=1}^p \frac{\partial \lambda}{\partial \theta_a} \frac{\partial \lambda}{\partial \theta_b} V_{\theta,ab} \tag{2.1}$$

and $\widehat{S} = S_{\widehat{\theta}}$ is the asymptotic estimate of the standard error.

2.3.2 Asymptotic Confidence Intervals for λ

If the distribution of $\widehat{T}$ were known, say $F(u) = \Pr(\widehat{T} \leq u)$, we would calculate the $\alpha/2$ and $1 - \alpha/2$ percentiles[2] of $\widehat{T}$, say u_α, $u_{1-\alpha/2}$. The interval

$$\widehat{I} = \left[\widehat{\lambda} - u_{1-\alpha/2}\widehat{S} \; ; \; \widehat{\lambda} - u_{\alpha/2}\widehat{S}\right]$$

would be a confidence interval for λ, with level $1 - \alpha$. In this case, the *coverage probability* of $\widehat{I}$, the probability that $\widehat{I}$ covers λ, would be $1 - \alpha$.

However, as we have seen in the preceding paragraph, we can only approximate, when n is sufficiently large, the distribution of $\widehat{T}$. Thus we use this approximation to calculate confidence intervals with coverage probability close to $1 - \alpha$.

Let $\mathcal{N}$ be a variate distributed as an $\mathcal{N}(0,1)$. Let ν_α be the α percentile of $\mathcal{N}$. From the result of Section 2.3.1, we can deduce a confidence interval for λ:

$$\widehat{I}_\mathcal{N} = \left[\widehat{\lambda} - \nu_{1-\alpha/2}\widehat{S}; \widehat{\lambda} + \nu_{1-\alpha/2}\widehat{S}\right]. \tag{2.2}$$

This interval is symmetric around $\widehat{\lambda}$ for $\nu_\alpha = -\nu_{1-\alpha}$.

The probability that $\widehat{T}$ is less than ν_α tends to α when n tends to infinity; the probability for λ to lie in $\widehat{I}_\mathcal{N}$ tends to $1 - \alpha$ when n tends to infinity. We say that $\widehat{I}_\mathcal{N}$ has *asymptotic level* $1 - \alpha$.

Remarks

1. By analogy to the Gaussian linear regression case, in the nonlinear regression model with homogeneous variance, we define an alternative confidence interval for λ. In Equation (2.2), we replace ν_α with $\sqrt{n/(n-p)}t_\alpha$, where t_α is the α percentile of a Student variate with $n - p$ degrees of freedom:

$$\widehat{I}_\mathcal{T} = \left[\widehat{\lambda} - \sqrt{\frac{n}{n-p}}t_{1-\alpha/2}\widehat{S}; \widehat{\lambda} + \sqrt{\frac{n}{n-p}}t_{1-\alpha/2}\widehat{S}\right]. \tag{2.3}$$

---

[2] The α percentile of a variate with distribution function F is the value of u, say u_α, such that $F(u_\alpha) = \alpha$ and $0 < \alpha < 1$.

$\widehat{I}_{\mathcal{T}}$ has the same asymptotic level as $\widehat{I}_{\mathcal{N}}$, but $\widehat{I}_{\mathcal{T}}$ is wider than $\widehat{I}_{\mathcal{N}}$ and its coverage probability will be greater. Some studies [HJM89] have shown that $\widehat{I}_{\mathcal{T}}$ has a coverage probability closer to $1 - \alpha$ than $\widehat{I}_{\mathcal{N}}$.

2. The intervals $\widehat{I}_{\mathcal{N}}$ and $\widehat{I}_{\mathcal{T}}$ are symmetric around $\widehat{\lambda}$. In some applications, a part of the symmetric confidence interval might not coincide with the set of variations of the parameter λ. For example, consider $\lambda = \exp \theta_3$ in the pasture regrowth example. If the estimate of the standard error of $\widehat{\lambda}$, say $\widehat{S}$, is bigger than $\widehat{\lambda}/\nu_{1-\alpha/2}$, then the lower bound of $\widehat{I}_{\mathcal{N}}$ is negative even though λ is strictly positive. In that case, it is easy to see that it is more appropriate to calculate a confidence interval for θ_3 and then to transform this interval taking the exponential of its limits to find a confidence interval for λ. More generally, let $\widehat{S}_3$ be the estimate of the standard error of $\widehat{\theta}_3$, and let g be a strictly increasing function of θ_3. If θ_3 lies in

$$\left[\widehat{\theta}_3 - \nu_{1-\alpha/2}\widehat{S}_3 ; \widehat{\theta}_3 + \nu_{1-\alpha/2}\widehat{S}_3 \right],$$

then $\lambda = g(\theta_3)$ lies in

$$\left[g(\widehat{\theta}_3 - \nu_{1-\alpha/2}\widehat{S}_3); g(\widehat{\theta}_3 + \nu_{1-\alpha/2}\widehat{S}_3) \right].$$

2.3.3 Asymptotic Tests of $\lambda = \lambda_0$ against $\lambda \neq \lambda_0$

Let λ_0 be a fixed value of λ and let the hypothesis of interest be H: $\lambda = \lambda_0$, against the alternative A: $\lambda \neq \lambda_0$.

Wald Test When H is true the limiting distribution of $(\widehat{\lambda} - \lambda_0)/\widehat{S}$ is an $\mathcal{N}(0,1)$. Thus, the limiting distribution of the test statistic

$$\mathcal{S}_{\mathrm{W}} = \frac{(\widehat{\lambda} - \lambda_0)^2}{\widehat{S}^2}$$

is a χ^2 with one degree of freedom. Hypothesis H will be rejected for large values of $\mathcal{S}_{\mathrm{W}}$, say $\mathcal{S}_{\mathrm{W}} > C$, where C is chosen such that $\Pr(Z_1 \leq C) = 1 - \alpha$, where Z_1 is distributed as a χ^2 with one degree of freedom.

This is the *Wald test*. When H is true, the probability for $\mathcal{S}_{\mathrm{W}}$ to be greater than C (in other words, the probability that hypothesis H is rejected when it should be accepted) tends to α when n tends to infinity. We say that this test has an *asymptotic error of the first kind*, equal to α. Assume now that H is false. Then the power of the test defined as the probability for $\mathcal{S}_{\mathrm{W}}$ to be greater than C (in other words, the probability to reject the hypothesis H when H is false) tends to 1 when n tends to infinity. We say that this test is consistent.

Remark As in Section 2.3.2, homogeneous variances can be considered separately; hypothesis H will be rejected if

$$\frac{n-p}{n}\mathcal{S}_W > C,$$

where C is chosen such that $\Pr(F_{1,n-p} \le C) = 1 - \alpha$, where $F_{1,n-p}$ is distributed as a Fisher variable with one and $n - p$ degrees of freedom.

Likelihood Ratio Test Another idea is to estimate the parameters under the constraint $\lambda = \lambda_0$, say $\widehat{\theta}_H$; then to estimate them without the constraint, say $\widehat{\theta}_A$; and then to compare the estimation criteria (1.10) $C(\widehat{\theta}_H)$ and $C(\widehat{\theta}_A)$ in the case of homogeneous variances. If H is true, the difference between $C(\widehat{\theta}_H)$ and $C(\widehat{\theta}_A)$ will be small. Let

$$\mathcal{S}_L = n \log C(\widehat{\theta}_H) - n \log C(\widehat{\theta}_A)$$

be the test statistic. When n tends to infinity, it can be shown that the limiting distribution of $\mathcal{S}_L$ is a χ^2 with one degree of freedom. Hypothesis H will be rejected when $\mathcal{S}_L > C$, where C is chosen such that $\Pr(Z_1 \le C) = 1 - \alpha$.

This test based on $\mathcal{S}_L$ is called a likelihood ratio test. It has the same asymptotic properties as the Wald test. Although the Wald test is easier to calculate, some theoretical arguments favor the likelihood ratio test.

2.3.4 Asymptotic Tests of $\Lambda\theta = L_0$ against $\Lambda\theta \ne L_0$

Let us return to Example 1.1.5 and assume that we want to test whether the parameters θ_2, θ_3, and θ_4 are identical. The hypothesis of interest is H: $\theta_2 = \theta_3 = \theta_4$, against the alternative that at least two of these parameters are different. H can be written as $\Lambda\theta = 0$, where Λ is the following 2×4 matrix:

$$\Lambda = \begin{pmatrix} 0 & 1 & -1 & 0 \\ 0 & 1 & 0 & -1 \end{pmatrix}. \tag{2.4}$$

The problems just defined can be solved by returning to the general case, with θ of dimension p. We aim to test the hypothesis H: $\Lambda\theta = L_0$ against A: $\Lambda\theta \ne L_0$, where Λ is a $q \times p$ matrix of rank q, $q < p$, and L_0 is a vector of dimension q. The model defined by hypothesis H is a model nested in the more general one defined by hypothesis A.

The Wald Test When H is true, the limiting distribution of

$$\mathcal{S}' = (\Lambda V_{\widehat{\theta}} \Lambda^T)^{-1/2}(\Lambda\widehat{\theta} - L_0)$$

is a q-dimensional Gaussian variable with mean 0 and covariance matrix equal to the $q \times q$ identity matrix. In these cases, the limiting distribution of the test statistic $\mathcal{S}_W = \sum_{a=1}^{q} \mathcal{S}_a'^2$ is a χ^2 with q degrees of freedom. The Wald test is defined by the rejection of H when $\mathcal{S}_W > C$, where $\Pr(Z_q \le C) = 1 - \alpha$ and Z_q is distributed as a χ^2 with q degrees of freedom.

Remark In the case of homogeneous variances, the test is defined by the rejection of H when

$$\frac{n-p}{n}\frac{S_W}{q} > C, \tag{2.5}$$

where C is chosen such that $\Pr(F_{q,n-p} \leq C) = 1 - \alpha$, where $F_{q,n-p}$ is distributed as a Fisher with q and $n-p$ degrees of freedom.

The Likelihood Ratio Test Let $\widehat{\theta}_H$ be the estimation of θ under the constraint $\Lambda\theta = L_0$; then, in the case of homogeneous variances, the limiting distribution of the test statistic $S_L = n \log C(\widehat{\theta}_H) - n \log C(\widehat{\theta}_A)$ is a χ^2 with q degrees of freedom. This result provides the likelihood ratio test.

Curve Comparison Let us return to Example 1.1.3, where we needed to compare two curves. The hypothesis of interest is H: $\theta_1^{May} = \theta_1^{June}$, $\theta_2^{May} = \theta_2^{June}$, $\theta_3^{May} = \theta_3^{June}$ against the alternative that at least one of these equalities is false. We create a data set by joining the data observed in May and June. We define the vector of parameters by joining θ^{May} and θ^{June}: Let

$$\theta = \begin{pmatrix} \theta^{May} \\ \theta^{June} \end{pmatrix}$$

be the $2p$ vector of parameters for the two curves. Then hypothesis H can be written as earlier $\Lambda\theta = 0$, where Λ is the following $3 \times 2p$ matrix:

$$\Lambda = \begin{pmatrix} 1 & 0 & 0 & 0 & -1 & 0 & 0 & 0 \\ 0 & 1 & 0 & 0 & 0 & -1 & 0 & 0 \\ 0 & 0 & 1 & 0 & 0 & 0 & -1 & 0 \end{pmatrix}. \tag{2.6}$$

As before, we define a test using the statistic S_W or S_L.

2.3.5 Bootstrap Estimations

Resampling methods like the jackknife and the *bootstrap* are especially useful for estimating the accuracy of an estimator. We observe $Y_1, Y_2, \ldots Y_n$; we choose a parametric nonlinear regression model with parameters θ, and we find an estimation procedure to estimate a function of θ, say $\lambda(\theta)$. We get $\widehat{\lambda} = \lambda(\widehat{\theta})$, but we are interested in calculating the accuracy of $\widehat{\lambda}$ or, more generally, in knowing its distribution (or some characteristics of it). If we were able to repeat the experiment under exactly the same conditions, we would observe $Y_1^1, Y_2^1, \ldots Y_n^1$, and in the same way as for $\widehat{\lambda}$ we would calculate $\widehat{\lambda}^1$. We could repeat it again and calculate $\widehat{\lambda}^2$ with $Y_1^2, Y_2^2, \ldots Y_n^2$. $\widehat{\lambda}^1, \widehat{\lambda}^2, \ldots$ would be a sample of random variables distributed as $\widehat{\lambda}$. This sample would approximate the distribution of $\widehat{\lambda}$. In short, resampling methods are a way to mimic the repetition of the experiment.

Bootstrap estimations are based on estimates $\widehat{\lambda}^\star = \lambda(\widehat{\theta}^\star)$ calculated from artificial bootstrap samples $(x_i, Y_{ij}^\star)$, $j = 1, \ldots, n_i$, $i = 1, \ldots k$, where

$$Y_{ij}^\star = f(x_i, \widehat{\theta}) + \varepsilon_{ij}^\star.$$

The errors $\varepsilon_{ij}^\star$ are simulated in the following way: Let $\widehat{\varepsilon}_{ij} = Y_{ij} - f(x_i, \widehat{\theta})$ be the residuals, and let $\widetilde{\varepsilon}_{ij} = \widehat{\varepsilon}_{ij} - \widehat{\varepsilon}_\bullet$, be the centered residuals, where $\widehat{\varepsilon}_\bullet$ is the sample mean, and $\widehat{\varepsilon}_\bullet = \sum_{i,j} \widehat{\varepsilon}_{ij}/n$. The set of $\varepsilon_{ij}^\star$, for $j = 1, \ldots n_i$, and $i = 1, \ldots k$ is a random sample from the empirical distribution function based on the $\widetilde{\varepsilon}_{ij}$ (n $\widetilde{\varepsilon}_{ij}$ are drawn with replacement, each with probability $1/n$). There are n^n such different samples.

$\widehat{\theta}^\star$ will be the value of θ that minimizes

$$C^\star(\theta) = \sum_{i=1}^{k} \sum_{j=1}^{n_i} (Y_{ij}^\star - f(x_i, \theta))^2.$$

The bootstrap estimate of λ is $\widehat{\lambda}^\star = \lambda(\widehat{\theta}^\star)$.

Let B be the number of bootstrap simulations. $(\widehat{\lambda}^{\star,b} = \lambda(\widehat{\theta}^{\star,b}), b = 1, \ldots, B)$ is a B *sample* of bootstrap estimates of λ. The choice of B will be discussed at the end of this section. The important result is that the distribution of $\widehat{\lambda}^\star$, estimated by the empirical[3] distribution function of the $(\widehat{\lambda}^{\star,b}, b = 1, \ldots B)$, approximates the distribution of $\widehat{\lambda}$. Let

$$\widehat{T}^\star = \frac{\widehat{\lambda}^\star - \widehat{\lambda}}{S_{\widehat{\theta}^\star}}.$$

Roughly speaking, the difference between the distribution functions of $\widehat{T}$ and $\widehat{T}^\star$ tends to 0 when the number of observations n is large; thus, we can use the quantiles of $\widehat{T}^\star$ instead of those of $\widehat{T}$ to construct confidence intervals or tests.

Let us emphasize that the bootstrap distribution for approximating the distribution of $\widehat{T}$ is theoretically justified when n is large and is an alternative to the centered normal distribution presented in Section 2.3.1. In real data sets, the number of observations is fixed and may be small. No theoretical result is known about the superiority of one of these approximations over the others.

Bootstrap Confidence Interval for λ

Let $(\widehat{T}^{\star,b}, b = 1, \ldots B)$ be a B sample of $\widehat{T}^\star$; $\widehat{T}^\star$ is calculated in the same way as $\widehat{T}$, replacing Y_{ij} with $Y_{ij}^\star$. Let b_α be the α percentile of the $\widehat{T}^{\star,b}$ (the way of calculating b_α is detailed in Section 2.4.1). It can be shown that $\Pr(\widehat{T} \leq b_\alpha)$ tends to α when n tends to infinity. This gives a *bootstrap confidence interval* for λ:

$$\widehat{I}_B = \left[\widehat{\lambda} - b_{1-\alpha/2}\widehat{S}; \widehat{\lambda} - b_{\alpha/2}\widehat{S} \right]. \tag{2.7}$$

For large n and B, the coverage probability of $\widehat{I}_B$ is close to $1 - \alpha$.

---

[3] Obviously, B must be large enough that the empirical distribution function is a good approximation of the distribution of $\widehat{\lambda}^\star$. If $B = n^n$, and if we draw all of the possible samples, we get the exact distribution of $\widehat{\lambda}^\star$.

Bootstrap Estimation of the Accuracy of $\widehat{\lambda}$

The variance, and even the bias, of $\widehat{\lambda}$ may be infinite or undefined. Nevertheless, their estimates (using the asymptotic results of Section 2.3.2 or the bootstrap) measure the localization and dispersion of the distribution of $\widehat{\lambda}$.

Variance The *bootstrap estimation of the variance* is calculated using the empirical variance of the B sample ($\widehat{\lambda}^{\star,b}$, $b = 1, \ldots, B$):

$$\widehat{S}^{\star 2} = \sum_{b=1}^{B} \frac{1}{B-1} \left(\widehat{\lambda}^{\star,b} - \widehat{\lambda}^{\star,\bullet} \right)^2, \tag{2.8}$$

where $\widehat{\lambda}^{\star,\bullet}$ is the sample mean $\widehat{\lambda}^{\star,\bullet} = \sum_{b=1}^{B} \widehat{\lambda}^{\star,b}/B$.

Bias As we noted in Section 2.3.2, the expectation of $\widehat{\lambda}$, $E(\widehat{\lambda})$, is close to λ when we have large values of n. In other words, the bias of $\widehat{\lambda}$, $BIAS = E(\widehat{\lambda}) - \lambda$, is close to 0. We can use the bootstrap sample to estimate this bias:

$$\widehat{BIAS}^{\star} = \widehat{\lambda}^{\star,\bullet} - \widehat{\lambda}. \tag{2.9}$$

Mean Square Error We can estimate the mean square error (MSE) in a similar way: $MSE = E(\widehat{\lambda} - \lambda)^2 = S^2 + BIAS^2$, where $S^2 = E(\widehat{\lambda} - E(\widehat{\lambda}))^2$ is the variance of $\widehat{\lambda}$; it is estimated by

$$\widehat{MSE}^{\star} = \widehat{S}^{\star 2} + \widehat{BIAS}^{\star 2}.$$

Median Because it is always defined, the median error, the median of $\widehat{\lambda} - \lambda$, is of special interest. Its bootstrap estimate, $\widehat{MED}^{\star}$, is the median of the B values $|\widehat{\lambda}^{\star,b} - \widehat{\lambda}|$.

Remarks

1. We have seen that the number of different bootstrap samples equals n^n. Obviously, we never choose for B a value that rapidly becomes unusable ($8^8 = 16,777,216$!). In practice, however, a moderate number usually suffices: If B is around 50, we can estimate the accuracy characteristic, and if B is around 200, we can calculate a confidence interval, for example.
2. Other resampling methods, like the jackknife, are available especially to estimate the accuracy characteristics (see [Wu86] and [Bun90] for details). These methods are less reliable than the bootstrap, however.
3. The bootstrap method in the case of heterogeneous variances is discussed in Section 3.4.3.

2.4 Applications

2.4.1 Pasture Regrowth: Calculation of a Confidence Interval for the Maximum Yield

Model The regression function is

$$f(x, \theta) = \theta_1 - \theta_2 \exp\left(-\exp(\theta_3 + \theta_4 \log x)\right),$$

and the variances are homogeneous: $\text{Var}(\varepsilon_i) = \sigma^2$.

Results

Parameters	Estimated Values	Asymptotic Covariance Matrix
θ_1	69.95	3.09
θ_2	61.68	3.87 6.66
θ_3	−9.209	0.76 1.25 0.37
θ_4	2.378	−0.22 −0.35 −0.09 0.027
σ^2	0.9306	

The parameter of interest is $\lambda(\theta) = \theta_1$.

Calculation of Confidence Intervals with Asymptotic Level 95%, Using Results of Section 2.3.2 , (d.f. is for degree of freedom):

$\widehat{\lambda}$	$\widehat{S}$	$\nu_{0.975}$	$\widehat{I}_{\mathcal{N}}$	$t_{0.975}$ (5 d.f.)	$\widehat{I}_{\mathcal{T}}$
69.95	1.76	1.96	[66.5 , 73.4]	2.57	[63.9 , 76.0]

d.f. is for degree of freedom

Calculation of Confidence Intervals with Asymptotic Level 95%, Using the Bootstrap Method Table 2.1 gives the estimated values of f, $\widehat{f}_i$, and the centered residuals $\widetilde{\varepsilon}_i$. For two bootstrap simulations, the table gives the bootstrap errors $\varepsilon_i^\star$, the bootstrap observations $Y_i^\star$, the bootstrap estimate of θ_1, and the corresponding asymptotic variance $S_{\widehat{\theta}^\star}$.

B, the number of bootstrap simulations, equals 199. The histogram of the $\widehat{T}^{\star,b}$, $b = 1, \ldots B$, is shown in Figure 2.1.

Calculation of the Percentiles of $(\widehat{T}^{\star,b}$, $b = 1, \ldots B)$ We calculate the 0.025 and 0.975 percentiles of the $\widehat{T}^{\star,b}$ as follows: Let $\widehat{T}^{\star,(b)}$ be the ordered values of $\widehat{T}^{\star,b}$ so that $\widehat{T}^{\star,(1)} \leq \widehat{T}^{\star,(2)} \leq \ldots \leq \widehat{T}^{\star,(199)}$; b_α is $\widehat{T}^{\star,(q_\alpha)}$, where q_α is the smallest integer such that q_α/B is greater than or equal to α. When $B = 199$, we find $b_{0.025} = \widehat{T}^{\star,(5)}$ and $b_{0.975} = \widehat{T}^{\star,(195)}$:

$\widehat{\lambda}$	$\widehat{S}$	$b_{0.025}$	$b_{0.975}$	$\widehat{I}_B$
69.95	1.76	−4.19	3.73	[63.4, 77.3]

We will see in Section 2.6 that in practice we use the function `quantile` of S-Plus.

Table 2.1. Results for two bootstrap simulations

$\widehat{f}_i$	$\widetilde{\varepsilon}_i$	$\varepsilon_i^{\star,1}$	$Y_i^{\star,1}$	$\varepsilon_i^{\star,2}$	$Y_i^{\star,2}$
9.411	−0.481	−0.481	8.93	−0.734	8.677
11.47	−0.669	−0.067	11.4	0.025	11.49
16.30	2.284	−0.734	15.57	−0.5	15.80
23.17	−0.843	0.025	23.20	−0.5	22.67
40.08	−0.734	−0.669	39.41	−0.481	39.60
56.18	−0.067	2.284	58.46	−0.669	55.51
60.74	0.986	0.025	60.77	−0.843	59.9
64.59	0.025	−0.734	63.86	−0.734	63.86
67.58	−0.5	2.284	69.86	2.284	69.86
$\widehat{\theta}_1 = 69.95$		$\widehat{\theta}_1^{\star,1} = 71.65$		$\widehat{\theta}_1^{\star,2} = 74.92$	
$\widehat{S} = 1.76$		$S_{\widehat{\theta}^{\star,1}} = 1.91$		$S_{\widehat{\theta}^{\star,2}} = 1.59$	

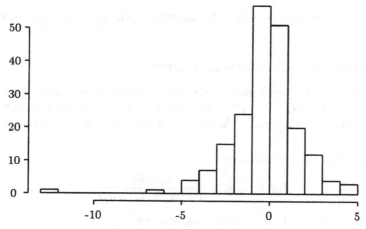

Figure 2.1. Pasture regrowth example: Histogram of $(\widehat{T}^{\star,b}, b = 1, \ldots B)$

Bootstrap Estimate of the Accuracy Characteristics:

$\widehat{\mathrm{BIAS}}^{\star}$	$\widehat{S}^{\star}$	$\widehat{\mathrm{MSE}}^{\star}$	$\widehat{\mathrm{MED}}^{\star}$
0.378 (0.5% of $\widehat{\theta}^1$)	2.30	5.42	69.78

2.4.2 Cortisol Assay: Estimation of the Accuracy of the Estimated Dose $\widehat{D}$

Model The regression function is

$$f(x, \theta) = \theta_1 + \frac{\theta_2 - \theta_1}{(1 + \exp(\theta_3 + \theta_4 x))^{\theta_5}},$$

and the variances are heterogeneous: $\mathrm{Var}(\varepsilon_i) = \sigma_i^2$.

Results

	Estimates	Asymptotic Covariance Matrix				
θ_1	133.30	0.727				
θ_2	2759.8	0.264	801			
θ_3	3.0057	−0.0137	−2.34	0.0338		
θ_4	3.1497	−0.00723	−2.33	0.0241	0.01845	
θ_5	0.64309	0.00341	0.568	−0.00714	−0.00516	0.00152

The parameter of interest is $D = \lambda(\theta) = 10^{f^{-1}(\mu,\theta)}$; see Equation (1.6), with $\mu = 2000$.

Calculation of Confidence Intervals with Asymptotic Level 95%, Using Results of Section 2.3.2

$\widehat{D}$	$\widehat{S}$	$\nu_{0.975}$	$\widehat{I}_{\mathcal{N}}$
0.0856	0.00175	1.96	[0.0822 , 0.0891]

We will discuss other methods for calculating the accuracy of $\widehat{D}$ in Chapter 5.

2.4.3 ELISA Test: Comparison of Curves

We want to test the *parallelism* of the response curves in order to estimate the difference $\beta = \theta_4^{\mathrm{May}} - \theta_4^{\mathrm{June}}$. We can do this by testing hypothesis H: $\Lambda\theta = 0$ against the alternative A: $\Lambda\theta \neq 0$, where Λ is the matrix defined by Equation (2.6),

Model The regression function is

$$f(x,\theta) = \theta_1 + \frac{\theta_2 - \theta_1}{1 + \exp\theta_3 (x - \theta_4)},$$

and the variances are homogeneous: $\mathrm{Var}(\varepsilon_i) = \sigma^2$.

Results

Estimated Values							
θ_1^{May}	θ_2^{May}	θ_3^{May}	θ_4^{May}	θ_1^{June}	θ_2^{June}	θ_3^{June}	θ_4^{June}
0.04279	1.936	2.568	3.467	0.0581	1.909	2.836	3.251
Asymptotic Covariance Matrix ($\times 10^4$)							
4.51							
−1.01	1.81						
15.2	−8.22	95.7					
−2.09	−0.502	−4.10	2.43				
0	0	0	0	2.51			
0	0	0	0	−0.647	1.92		
0	0	0	0	10.5	−8.74	106	
0	0	0	0	−1.05	−0.727	−0.988	1.83

$\widehat{\sigma}^2 = 0.0005602.$

Wald Test of H: $\Lambda\theta = 0$ against A: $\Lambda\theta \neq 0$. See Section2.3.3.

The value of the Wald test is $S_W = 4.53$. This number must be compared to 7.8, which is the 0.95 quantile of a χ^2 with three degrees of freedom. The hypothesis of *parallelism* is not rejected.

Because the variance of errors is constant, we can compare

$$\frac{n-p}{n}\frac{S_W}{q} = \frac{32-8}{32}\frac{7.8}{3} = 1.133$$

to 3, which is the 0.95 quantile of a Fisher with 3 and 24 degrees of freedom.

Likelihood ratio tests See Section2.3.3.

The two first columns of Table 2.2 show the estimated parameters under A and under the constraints defined by H and the corresponding values of the sum of squares C.

Table 2.2. ELISA test example: Estimated parameters under hypothesis A, the *parallelism* is not verified; hypothesis H, the curves are *parallel*; and the hypothesis that $\beta = 0$

	Under A	Under H	Under $\beta = 0$
θ_1^{May}	0.0428	0.0501	0.0504
θ_2^{May}	1.936	1.924	1.926
θ_3^{May}	2.568	2.688	2.635
θ_4^{May}	3.467	3.470	3.356
θ_1^{June}	0.058	0.0501	0.0504
θ_2^{June}	1.909	1.924	1.926
θ_3^{June}	2.836	2.688	2.635
θ_4^{June}	3.251	3.247	3.356
$C(\theta)$	0.0179	0.0206	0.183

The test statistic $S_L = 32 * (\log(0.0206) - \log(0.0179))$ equals 4.5. Thus, hypothesis H is not rejected.

The estimated value of $\beta = \theta_4^{May} - \theta_4^{June}$ is $\widehat{\beta} = 0.223$. We can carry out a likelihood ratio test by comparing $C(\widehat{\theta}_H)$ with $C(\widehat{\theta}_{\beta=0})$, which is the sum of squares when the parameters are estimated under the constraint $\beta = 0$; see the third column of Table 2.2. $S_L = 32 * (\log(0.183) - \log(0.0206)) = 69.9$. This number must be compared to 3.8, the 0.95 quantile of a χ^2 with one degree of freedom. The hypothesis $\beta = 0$ is rejected.

Conclusion of the Test In this experiment, we conclude that the *potency ρ* of the serum taken in June *relative* to the serum taken in May is estimated by $\widehat{\rho} = 10^{-\widehat{\beta}} = 0.59$ and that ρ is significantly different from 1.

Calculation of a Confidence Interval for ρ The parameter of interest is $\rho = \lambda(\theta) = 10^{\theta_4^{June} - \theta_4^{May}}$.

Calculation of Confidence Intervals with Asymptotic Level 95%, Using Results of Section 2.3.2 (d.f. is for degree of freedom):

$\widehat{\rho}$	$\widehat{S}$	$\nu_{0.975}$	$\widehat{I}_{\mathcal{N}}$	$t_{0.975}$ (27 d.f.)	$\widehat{I}_{\mathcal{T}}$
0.59	0.0192	1.96	[0.561 , 0.636]	2.05	[0.555 , 0.642]

$\widehat{I}_{\mathcal{T}}$ is not much different from $\widehat{I}_{\mathcal{N}}$ because $n - p$ is large, $n/(n - p)$ is close to 1, and the difference between ν_α and t_α is small.

Calculation of Confidence Intervals with Asymptotic Level 95%, Using the Bootstrap Method The number of bootstrap simulations is $B = 199$. The histogram of the $\widehat{T}^{\star,b}$, $b = 1, \ldots B$, is shown in Figure 2.2.

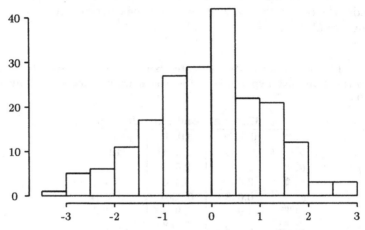

Figure 2.2. ELISA test example: Histogram of $(\widehat{T}^{\star,b}, b = 1, \ldots B)$

The results follow:

$\widehat{\rho}$	$\widehat{S}$	$b_{0.025}$	$b_{0.975}$	$\widehat{I}_B$
0.59	0.0192	−2.61	2.17	[0.557 , 0.649]

In this example, the bootstrap shows that $\widehat{I}_B$ is longer than $\widehat{I}_{\mathcal{N}}$ but is nearly equal to $\widehat{I}_{\mathcal{T}}$. Moreover, the bootstrap estimation of the standard error of $\widehat{\rho}$ is $\widehat{S}^\star = 0.0199$. The differences between the methods are not very important from a practical point of view.

2.4.4 Ovocytes: Calculation of Confidence Regions

Although this experiment tested several cryoprotectants in different experimental conditions (with or without treatment, at several temperatures) and yielded 15 curves to be estimated and compared, we present here the results for only two curves. We compute two types of confidence regions: Confidence ellipsoids and likelihood contours.

Confidence Ellipsoids Let θ be the pair (P_w, P_s). When the number of observations tends to infinity, the limiting distribution of

$$S'(\theta) = V_{\widehat{\theta}}^{-1/2}(\widehat{\theta} - \theta)$$

is a standard two dimensional normal distribution $\mathcal{N}(0, I_2)$, or the limiting distribution of

$$S_W(\theta) = S_1'^2 + S_2'^2$$

is a χ^2 with two degrees of freedom. Let $r_\alpha(2)$ be the α percentile of a χ^2 with two degrees of freedom, and let $\mathcal{R}_W$ be the set of θ such that $S_W(\theta) \leq r_{1-\alpha}(2)$. $\mathcal{R}_W$ is an ellipse that covers θ with probability close to $1 - \alpha$.

Likelihood Contours Constructing confidence ellipses is based on the limiting distribution of $\widehat{\theta} - \theta$. Another way to calculate confidence regions for θ is to consider the limiting distribution of the statistic

$$S_L(\theta) = n \log C(\theta) - n \log C(\widehat{\theta}).$$

$S_L(\theta)$ is a χ^2 with two degrees of freedom. Let $\mathcal{R}_L$ be the set of θ such that $S_L(\theta) \leq r_{1-\alpha}(2)$. $\mathcal{R}_L$ is a region of the plane that covers θ with probability close to $1 - \alpha$.

Figure 2.3 illustrates the confidence ellipses and the likelihood contours with level 95% for the parameters (P_w, P_s) in Example 1.1.4. In this example, the likelihood contours are close to the ellipses, but we will see that this is not always the case. In fact, the discrepancy between these regions is related to the discrepancy between the distribution of $\widehat{\theta} - \theta$ and its approximation by a centered Gaussian variable.

Remarks When p, the dimension of θ, is greater than 2, the confidence ellipsoids for θ are defined by the set of θ such that $S_W(\theta) \leq r_{1-\alpha}(p)$, where $r_\alpha(p)$ is the α percentile of a χ^2 with p degrees of freedom. Usually the sections of the regions are drawn in two dimensions, and they give conditional information. Consider the case $p = 3$. The sections of the confidence regions in the plane (θ_1, θ_2) are the sets of (θ_1, θ_2) such that $S_W(\theta_1, \theta_2, \widehat{\theta}_3) \leq r_{1-\alpha}(3)$.

2.4.5 Isomerization: An Awkward Example

Model The regression function is

$$f(x, \theta) = \frac{\theta_1 \theta_3 (P - I/1.632)}{1 + \theta_2 H + \theta_3 P + \theta_4 I},$$

and the variances are homogeneous: $\text{Var}(\varepsilon_i) = \sigma^2$.

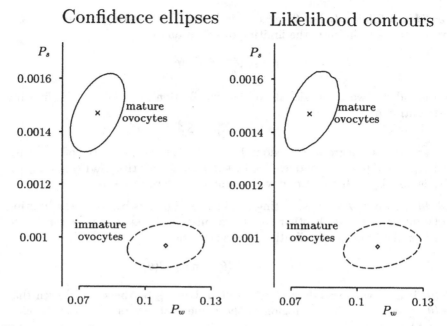

Figure 2.3. Ovocytes example: 95% confidence ellipses and likelihood contours for the parameters (P_w, P_s)

Table 2.3. Isomerization example: Estimated parameters and standard errors, normal confidence intervals

	Estimates	Standard Errors $(\widehat{S})$	95% Confidence Interval $\widehat{I}_\mathcal{N}$
θ_1	35.9193	7.49	[21.20 50.60]
θ_2	0.0708583	0.163	[−0.249 0.391]
θ_3	0.0377385	0.0913	[−0.141 0.217]
θ_4	0.167166	0.379	[−0.577 0.911]
σ^2	0.13477		

Calculation of Confidence Intervals Using the Percentiles of a Gaussian Distribution for Each Parameter The estimated values of the parameters and their standard errors and of the confidence intervals calculated using Equation (2.2) are given in Table 2.3.

The standard errors are so large for parameters θ_2, θ_3, and θ_4 that the value 0 is inside the confidence intervals. Obviously, the hypothesis $\theta_2 = \theta_3 = \theta_4 = 0$ is meaningless. Figure 2.4 illustrates the discrepancy between the distribution of $\widehat{\theta} - \theta$ and its approximation by the distribution $\mathcal{N}(0, V_\theta)$. In this figure, the sections of the confidence ellipsoids and likelihood contours in the plane (θ_1, θ_2) clearly differ significantly in their appearance. Thus, we cannot use the percentiles of a Gaussian distribution to calculate the confidence intervals. Instead, let us try the bootstrap method.

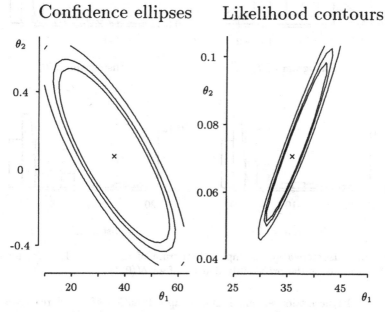

Figure 2.4. Isomerization example: The confidence ellipses and likelihood contours for the parameters (θ_1, θ_2) are drawn at levels 90%, 95%, and 99%

Calculation of Confidence Intervals Using the Bootstrap Method $B = 199$ bootstrap simulations have been done to calculate another approximation of the distribution of $\widehat{\theta}$. Let

$$\widehat{T}_a = \frac{\widehat{\theta}_a - \theta_a}{\widehat{S}_a},$$

where θ_a is the component a of θ and $\widehat{S}_a$ is the estimation of the standard error of $\widehat{\theta}_a$. For each parameter, the bootstrap estimation of the distribution of $\widehat{T}_a$ is shown in Figure 2.5. Note that the bootstrap distributions are very far from the Gaussian distribution, except for the first parameter.

Bootstrap Estimations of Standard Error and Bias for Each Parameter Estimator The results are Table 2.4.

The bootstrap estimations of the standard errors, $\widehat{S}_a^*$ (see Equation (2.8)), are of the same magnitude as $\widehat{S}_a$. The bootstrap yields a high value of the bias (see Equation (2.9)) for θ_1, but the bias is small for the other parameters. The 0.025 and 0.975 percentiles of the $\widehat{T}_a^{*,b}$ ($\widehat{T}_a^*$ is the bootstrap version of $\widehat{T}_a$) are calculated as in Section 2.4.1. They show the asymmetry of the estimators' distribution. By comparison, the 0.025 percentile of a Gaussian $\mathcal{N}(0, 1)$

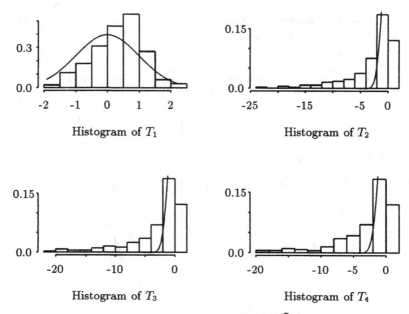

Figure 2.5. Isomerization example: Histogram of $(\widehat{T}^{*,b},\ b = 1, \ldots B)$ for each parameter; the line is the probability density of an $\mathcal{N}(0, 1)$

Table 2.4. Isomerization example: Bootstrap estimation of standard errors and bias for the parameters θ; 2.5% and 97.5% percentiles of the bootstrap distribution of $\widehat{T}$; bootstrap confidence intervals for the θ

	$\widehat{S}^*$	$\widehat{BIAS}^*$ (% of bias)	$b_{0.025}$	$b_{0.975}$	$\widehat{I}_B$
θ_1	9.83	5.47 (15)	-1.38	1.69	[23.2 46.2]
θ_2	0.133	0.002 (3)	-15.2	0.137	[0.048 2.56]
θ_3	0.080	0.002 (6)	-16.4	0.151	[0.024 1.54]
θ_4	0.322	0.008 (5)	-15.4	0.144	[0.112 6.05]

distribution is $\nu_{0.975} = 1.96$. The last column gives the bootstrap confidence intervals (see Equation 2.7). For the three last parameters the lower bound of the intervals is positive; this condition is more realistic than the negative bounds obtained with $\widehat{I}_N$. The confidence intervals are not symmetric around the estimated values $\widehat{\theta}_a$.

Calculation of Confidence Intervals Using a New Parameterization of the Function f An alternative to the bootstrap is to find another parameterization of the function $f(x, \theta)$ that reduces the discrepancy between the distribution of $\widehat{T}$ and the approximation of $\widehat{T}$ by a Gaussian distribution.

Model A new parameterization, suggested by several authors (see [BW88], for example) is defined by considering a new set of parameters, say $(\beta_1, \beta_2, \beta_3, \beta_4)$.

These are obtained by eliminating the product $\theta_1\theta_3$ in Equation (1.9). The model function is now defined by

$$f(x,\beta) = \frac{P - I/1.632}{\beta_1 + \beta_2 H + \beta_3 P + \beta_4 I}, \tag{2.10}$$

and $\mathrm{Var}(\varepsilon_i) = \sigma^2$.

Table 2.5. Isomerization example with the new parameterization: Estimated parameters and standard errors; normal confidence intervals

	Estimates	Standard Errors $(\widehat{S})$	95% Confidence Interval $\widehat{I}_N$
β_1	0.73738	1.66	[-2.51 3.98]
β_2	0.052274	0.00418	[0.0441 0.0605]
β_3	0.027841	0.00581	[0.0164 0.0392]
β_4	0.12331	0.0161	[0.0917 0.155]
σ^2	0.13477		

Parameter and Standard Error Estimations The results are given in Table 2.5. The estimated accuracy of the parameters is reasonable, and the discrepancy between confidence ellipses and likelihood contours for the pair (β_1, β_2) is not as big as for the pair (θ_1, θ_2); see Figure 2.6.

Let us assume that we are interested in calculating confidence intervals for the parameters θ. We want to calculate confidence intervals for each θ_a using the confidence regions calculated for β. In our example, the relations between θ and β are easy to write:

$$\theta_1 = 1/\beta_3,$$
$$\theta_2 = \beta_2/\beta_1,$$
$$\theta_3 = \beta_3/\beta_1,$$
$$\theta_4 = \beta_4/\beta_1.$$

If β_3 lies in the interval $[0.0164, 0.0392]$, then θ_1 lies in $[25.5, 60.8]$; however, we see that the same reasoning cannot be applied to θ_2, because 0 lies in the confidence interval for β_1. Thus, in this example, the calculation of a confidence interval for the parameters θ_a, $a = 1, \ldots p$, is only possible for θ_1. Only the bootstrap method allows us to calculate confidence intervals for each parameter.

2.4.6 Pasture Regrowth: Calculation of a Confidence Interval for $\lambda = \exp\theta_3$

Let us return to our pasture regrowth example to illustrate how to calculate a confidence interval that respects the constraint that parameter λ must be positive.

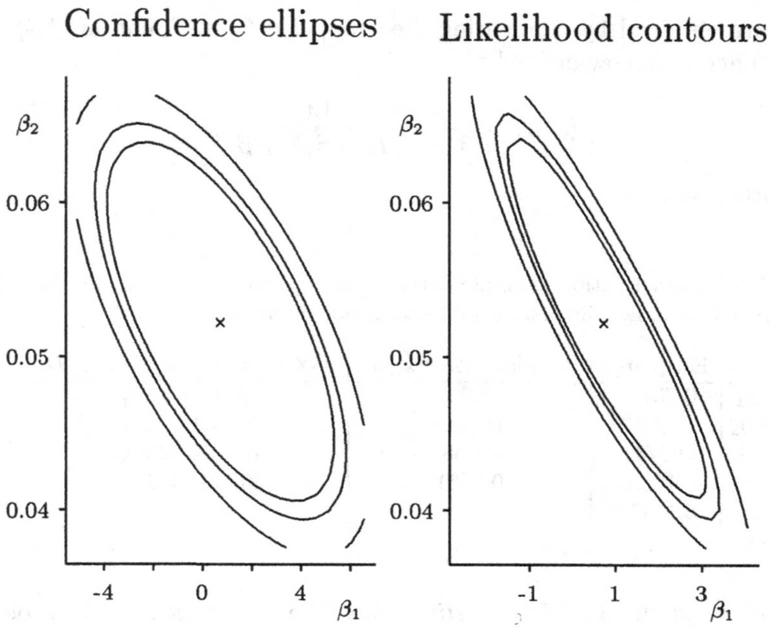

Confidence ellipses   Likelihood contours

Figure 2.6. Isomerization example: The confidence ellipses and likelihood contours for the parameters (β_1, β_2) are drawn at levels 90%, 95%, and 99%

Model The regression function is

$$f(x, \theta) = \theta_1 - \theta_2 \exp\left(-\exp(\theta_3 + \theta_4 \log x)\right),$$

and the variances are homogeneous: $\mathrm{Var}(\varepsilon_i) = \sigma^2$.

Results

Parameters	Estimated Values	Asymptotic Covariance Matrix			
θ_1	69.95	3.09			
θ_2	61.68	3.87	6.66		
θ_3	−9.209	0.76	1.25	0.37	
θ_4	2.378	−0.22	−0.35	−0.09	0.027
σ^2	0.9306				

The parameter of interest is $\lambda(\theta) = \exp \theta_3$.

Calculation of Confidence Intervals with Asymptotic Level 95%, Using Results of Section 2.3.2

$\widehat{\lambda}$	$\widehat{S}$	$\nu_{0.975}$	$\widehat{I_N}$
0.0001001	0.0000609	1.96	$[-.0000194, .000219]$

It is immediately apparent that this confidence interval is unusable because λ cannot be negative. The result would have been the same if we had estimated λ by replacing the model function (1.1) with the following one: $f(x, \theta_1, \theta_2, \lambda, \theta_4) = \theta_1 - \theta_2 \exp(-\lambda x^{\theta_4})$.

Another way to calculate a confidence interval for λ is to transform the confidence interval calculated for θ_3. If θ_3 lies in $[-10.4 \ -8.01]$, then $\lambda = \exp \theta_3$ lies in $[0.0000303 \ , \ 0.000331]$. By construction, this confidence interval is adapted to the set of variation of λ.

2.5 Conclusion

We have proposed several methods to estimate confidence intervals based on approximating the distribution of $\widehat{\lambda}$ by either the Gaussian distribution or the bootstrap distribution. In some cases (see Example 2.4.1), it is more convenient to consider a monotone transformation of the parameter of interest in place of the parameter itself, because the distribution of its estimator is better approximated by a Gaussian distribution. In other cases, the bootstrap method is more appropriate (see Example 2.4.5). The examples treated in this chapter show that there is no rule to decide in advance which is the correct method. Nevertheless, in each case, the final choice was based on the adequacy of the result and the nature of the parameter of interest.

2.6 Using nls2

This section reproduces the commands and files used in this chapter to analyze the examples using **nls2**. It is assumed that the commands introduced in Section 1.6 have already been executed.

Pasture Regrowth Example: Confidence Interval for the Maximum Yield

The results of estimation have been stored in the structure `pasture.nl1` (see Section 1.6, page 19). Now we want to calculate a confidence interval for the maximum yield, the parameter θ_1.

Confidence Interval for $\lambda = \theta_1$ with Asymptotic Level 95%

We use the function `confidence`. This function calculates the confidence interval $\widehat{I}_N$ defined by Equation (2.2), page 32, and the confidence interval $\widehat{I}_T$ defined by Equation (2.3), page 32. By default, the asymptotic level is 95%.

```
> pasture.conf.par <- confidence(pasture.nl1)
```

We display the values of $\widehat{\lambda}$, $\widehat{S}$, $\nu_{0.975}$, $\widehat{I}_N$, $t_{0.975}$ (five degrees of freedom), and $\widehat{I}_T$:

```
> cat("Estimated value of lambda:", pasture.conf.par$psi[1],"\n" )
> cat("Estimated value of S:",pasture.conf.par$std.error[1],"\n" )
> cat("nu_(0.975):", qnorm(0.975),"\n" )
> cat("Estimated value of In:",
        pasture.conf.par$normal.conf.int[1,],"\n" )
> cat("t_(0.975, 5):", qt(0.975,5),"\n" )
> cat("Estimated value of It:",
        pasture.conf.par$student.conf.int[1,],"\n" )
```

Confidence Interval for $\lambda = \theta_1$ Using Bootstrap with Asymptotic Level 95%

To calculate the confidence interval $\widehat{I}_B$ defined by Equation (2.7), page 36, we use the function **bootstrap**. Several methods of bootstrap simulation are possible. Here, we choose **residuals**, which means that pseudoerrors are randomly generated among the centered residuals.

To initialize the iterative process of **bootstrap**, **nls2** must be called with the option **renls2**. We also set the option **control** so that intermediary results are not printed. Finally, we call the function **delnls2** to destroy any internal structures:

```
> pasture.nl1 <- nls2(pasture, "pasture.mod1",
            list(theta.start= c(70, 60, 0, 1), max.iters=100),
            control=list(freq=0),
            renls2=T)
> pasture.boot <- bootstrap(pasture.nl1,
            method="residuals",
            n.loops=199)
> delnls2()
```

We calculate the values of $\widehat{T}^{\star,b}$, $b = 1, \ldots 199$ (see Section 2.3.5) and illustrate their distribution function by plotting them in a histogram (see Figure 2.1, page 39):

```
> P1.B <- pasture.boot$pStar[,1]
> SE.P1.B <- sqrt(pasture.boot$var.pStar[,1])
> T.B <- (P1.B-pasture.nl1$theta[1])/SE.P1.B
> hist(T.B,nclass=12,
        title="Pasture regrowth example",
        sub="Histogram of bootstrap estimations for T")
```

We calculate the 0.0025 and 0.975 percentiles of the $\widehat{T}^{\star,b}$, $b_{0.025}$ and $b_{0.975}$ (see Section 2.4.1) using the function **quantile** of S-Plus, and we display the values of $\widehat{\lambda}$, $\widehat{S}$, $b_{0.025}$, $b_{0.975}$, and $\widehat{I}_B$:

```
>    # Print the results:
> cat("Estimated value of lambda:", pasture.nl1$theta[1],"\n")
> cat("Estimated value of S:",coef(pasture.nl1)$std.error[1],"\n")
> qu   <- quantile(T.B,probs=c(0.975,0.025))
> cat("b_(0.025):", qu[2],"\n" )
```

```
> cat("b_(0.975):", qu[1],"\n" )
> cat("Estimated value of Ib:",
    pasture.nl1$theta[1]+qu[2]*coef(pasture.nl1)$std.error[1],
    pasture.nl1$theta[1]+qu[1]*coef(pasture.nl1)$std.error[1],"\n")
```

Finally, we calculate the accuracy characteristics of the bootstrap estimation: the bias ($\widehat{\mathrm{BIAS}}^*$; Equation (2.9)), the variance ($\widehat{S}^*$; Equation (2.8)), the mean square error ($\widehat{\mathrm{MSE}}^*$), and the median ($\widehat{\mathrm{MED}}^*$):

```
> cat("BIAS:" , (mean(P1.B)-pasture.nl1$theta[1]),"\n" )
> cat("S:" ,sqrt(var(P1.B)),"\n" )
> cat("MSE:" ,
    var(P1.B)+(mean(P1.B)-pasture.nl1$theta[1])^2 ,"\n" )
> cat("MED:" ,median(P1.B) ,"\n" )
```

Note: The bootstrap method generates different numbers on each execution. Thus, results of these commands may vary slightly from those displayed in Section 2.4.1, page 38.

Cortisol Assay Example: Confidence Interval for D

We calculated an estimate of the calibration curve (see Section 1.6, page 21) in structure **corti.nl1**, and now we want to calculate a confidence interval for the estimation of the dose of hormone D contained in a preparation that has the expected response $\mu = 2000$ c.p.m.

Confidence Interval for D

We describe the function D in a file called **corti.D**. The expected response μ is introduced by the key word **pbispsi**:

```
psi D;
ppsi n,d,a,b,g;
pbispsi mu;
aux X1, X2, X;
subroutine;
begin
X1 = log((d-n)/(mu-n));
X2 = exp(X1/g);
X = (log(X2-1)-a)/b;
D = 10**X;
end
```

To calculate a confidence interval for D, we apply the **confidence** function. Then we display the results of interest, $\widehat{D}$, $\widehat{S}$, $\nu_{0.975}$, and $\widehat{I}_{\mathcal{N}}$:

```
> loadnls2(psi="")
> corti.conf.D <- confidence(corti.nl1,file="corti.D",pbispsi=2000)
>    # Print the results:
```

```
> cat("Estimated value of D:", corti.conf.D$psi,"\n" )
> cat("Estimated value of S:",corti.conf.D$std.error,"\n" )
> cat("nu_(0.975):", qnorm(0.975),"\n" )
> cat("Estimated value of In:",corti.conf.D$normal.conf.int,"\n" )
```

(The results are given in Section 2.4.2, page 39.)

ELISA Test Example: Comparison of Curves

The results of estimation have been stored in the structure `elisa.nl1` (see Section 1.6, page 22). Now we want to test the *parallelism* of the May and June curves.

Wald Test with Asymptotic Level 95%

To test the parallelism of the response curves with a Wald test (see Section 2.3.3), we use the function `wald`.

First we describe the functions to be tested in a file called `elisa.wald`:

```
psi d1,d2,d3;
ppsi p1_c1, p2_c1, p3_c1, p1_c2, p2_c2, p3_c2;
subroutine;
begin
d1=p1_c1-p1_c2;
d2=p2_c1-p2_c2;
d3=p3_c1-p3_c2;
end
```

We apply the function `wald` and display the value of the statistic S_W and the 0.95 quantile of a χ^2 with three degrees of freedom from which it should be compared:

```
> elisa.wald <- wald(elisa.nl1,file="elisa.wald")
>    # Print the results:
> cat("SW:",elisa.wald$statistic,"\n" )
> cat("X2(3):", qchisq(0.95, 3),"\n" )
```

Because the variances are homogeneous, we calculate the test statistic defined in Equation (2.5), page 35:

```
> SF <- (elisa.wald$statistic*(32-8))/(32*3)
> cat("SF:", SF,"\n" )
> cat("F(3,24):", qf(0.95, 3,24), "\n" )
```

Likelihood Ratio Tests

To test the parallelism of the curves by likelihood ratio tests (see Section 2.3.3), we have to estimate the parameters under hypothesis A (*the parallelism of the curves is not verified*), under hypothesis H (*the curves are parallel*), and under the last hypothesis (*the curves are identical*).

Estimation under hypothesis A has already been calculated: A is the hypothesis under which structure `elisa.nl1` has been built.

Estimation under hypothesis H is done by setting equality constraints on all of the parameters except for the last one. Equality constraints are given with the option `eqp.theta`:

```
> elisa.nlH <- nls2(elisa,
    list(file="elisa.mod1", eqp.theta=c(1,2,3,4,1,2,3,5)),
    rep(c(2,0,1,0),2))
```

Estimation under the last hypothesis is done by setting equality constraints on all of the parameters:

```
> elisa.nlb <- nls2(elisa,
    list(file="elisa.mod1", eqp.theta=c(1,2,3,4,1,2,3,4)),
    rep(c(2,0,1,0),2))
```

We display the estimated values of the parameters and the sums of squares for the three hypothesis:

```
> cat("Estimated values of the parameters for the 3 hypothesis:\n")
> print(elisa.nl1$theta)
> print(elisa.nlH$theta)
> print(elisa.nlb$theta)
> cat("Estimated sums of squares for the 3 hypothesis:\n",
    elisa.nl1$rss, "\n", elisa.nlH$rss,"\n",
    elisa.nlb$rss,"\n")
```

Now, we calculate the test statistic S_L and display the 0.95 quantile of a χ^2 with one degree of freedom from which they should be compared. We also print the estimated value of $\beta = (\theta_4^{May} - \theta_4^{June})$:

```
> cat("Sl:",
    32*(log(elisa.nlH$rss) - log(elisa.nl1$rss)),
    32*(log(elisa.nlb$rss) - log(elisa.nlH$rss)),"\n" )
> cat("X2(0.95,1):", qchisq(0.95,1),"\n" )
> cat("Estimated value of beta:",
    elisa.nlH$theta["p4_c1"] - elisa.nlH$theta["p4_c2"],"\n" )
```

Confidence Interval for ρ with Asymptotic Level 95%

Now we want to calculate a confidence interval for a function of the parameters: $\rho = \lambda(\theta) = 10^{(\theta_4^{June} - \theta_4^{May})}$.

We describe ρ in a file called `elisa.ro`:

```
psi ro;
ppsi p4_c1, p4_c2;
subroutine;
begin
ro=10**(p4_c2-p4_c1);
end
```

The function `confidence` is applied to the structure `elisa.nlH`, which contains the results of estimation under hypothesis H (*the curves are parallel*). We display the values of $\hat{\rho}$, the standard error $(\hat{S})$, $\nu_{0.975}$, $\hat{I}_{\mathcal{N}}$, $t_{0.975}$ (27 degrees of freedom), and $\hat{I}_{\mathcal{T}}$:

```
> elisa.ro <- confidence(elisa.nlH, file="elisa.ro")
>    # Print the results:
> cat("Estimated value of rho:", elisa.ro$psi,"\n" )
> cat("Estimated value of S:",elisa.ro$std.error,"\n" )
> cat("nu_(0.975):", qnorm(0.975),"\n" )
> cat("Estimated value of In:",elisa.ro$normal.conf.int,"\n" )
> cat("t_(0.975, 27):", qt(0.975,27),"\n" )
> cat("Estimated value of It:",elisa.ro$student.conf.int,"\n" )
```

Confidence Interval for ρ Using Bootstrap with Asymptotic Level 95%

To calculate confidence intervals for ρ with bootstrap simulations (see Section 2.3.5, page 35) we apply the function `bootstrap`.

To initialize the iterative bootstrap process, `nls2` is first called with the option `renls2`, and, finally, the function `delnls2` cleans the internal structures:

```
> elisa.nlH <- nls2(elisa,
    list(file="elisa.mod1", eqp.theta=c(1,2,3,4,1,2,3,5)),
    rep(c(2,0,1,0),2),
    control=list(freq=0),
    renls2=T)
> elisa.boot.ro <- bootstrap(elisa.nlH,method="residuals",
                    file="elisa.ro", n.loops=199)
> delnls2()
```

We display the values of $\hat{\rho}$, $\hat{S}$, $b_{0.025}$, $b_{0.975}$, and $\hat{I}_B$:

```
> cat("Estimated value of rho:",elisa.ro$psi,"\n" )
> cat("Estimated value of S:", elisa.ro$std.error,"\n" )
> qu  <- quantile((elisa.boot.ro$tStar,probs=c(0.975,0.025))
> cat("b_(0.025):", qu[2],"\n" )
> cat("b_(0.975):", qu[1],"\n" )
> cat("Estimated value of Ib:", elisa.boot.ro$conf.int ,"\n" )
> cat("Bootstrap standard error:", sqrt(var(elisa.boot.ro$psiStar))
```

To illustrate the distribution function of $\hat{T}^\star$, we plot a histogram of their values (see Figure 2.2, page 42):

```
> hist(elisa.boot.ro$tStar, nclass=9,
        title="ELISA example",
        sub="Histogram of bootstrap estimations for T")
```

Note: The bootstrap method generates different numbers on each execution. Thus, results of these commands may vary slightly from those displayed in Section 2.4.3, page 40.

Ovocytes Example

Confidence Ellipsoids and Likelihood Contours for the Parameters (P_w, P_s)

The results of estimation by **nls2** have been stored in the structure **ovo.nl1** (see Section 1.6, page 25). We want to compare the parameters P_w and P_s by calculating confidence ellipsoids and likelihood contours in the space of these parameters.

The functions **ellips** and **iso** are used. **ellips** returns what is necessary to plot confidence ellipsoids, and **iso** returns what is necessary to define confidence regions in a two-dimensional space of parameters. The plots themselves are drawn by the graphical functions of S-Plus:

```
> ovo.ell1 <- ellips(ovo.nl1, axis=c("Pw_c1","Ps_c1"))
> ovo.ell2 <- ellips(ovo.nl1, axis=c("Pw_c2","Ps_c2"))
> ovo.iso1 <- iso(ovo.nl1, axis=c("Pw_c1","Ps_c1"))
> ovo.iso2 <- iso(ovo.nl1, axis=c("Pw_c2","Ps_c2"))
>     # Graphical functions of Splus
> par(mfrow=c(1,2))
> plot(x=c(.06,.13),y=c(0.0008,.0017),type="n",xlab="Pw",ylab="Ps")
> contour(ovo.ell1,levels=qchisq(0.95,2),add=T,labex=0)
> contour(ovo.ell2,levels=qchisq(0.95,2),add=T,labex=0)
> text(0.1,0.0015,"mature ovocytes")
> text(0.08,0.001,"immature ovocytes")
> title("Confidence ellipses")
> plot(x=c(.06,.13),y=c(0.0008,.0017),type="n",xlab="Pw",ylab="Ps")
> contour(ovo.iso1,levels=qchisq(0.95,2),add=T,labex=0)
> contour(ovo.iso2,levels=qchisq(0.95,2),add=T,labex=0)
> text(0.095,0.0015,"mature ovocytes")
> text(0.08,0.001,"immature ovocytes")
> title("Likelihood contours")
```

(See Figure 2.3, page 44.)

Isomerization Example

We have calculated one estimate of the parameters (see Section 1.6, page 26) in the structure **isomer.nl1**, and now we want to calculate confidence intervals for each parameter.

Confidence Intervals for Each Parameter with Asymptotic Level 95%

We use the function `confidence` to calculate the confidence interval $\widehat{I}_N$ defined by Equation (2.2), page 32, for each parameter:

```
> isomer.conf.par <- confidence(isomer.nl1)
```

We display the estimated values of the parameters, their standard errors $(\widehat{S})$, and the confidence interval $\widehat{I}_N$:

```
> print(matrix(c(isomer.conf.par$psi,
                 isomer.conf.par$std.error,
                 isomer.conf.par$normal.conf.int[,"lower"],
                 isomer.conf.par$normal.conf.int[,"upper"]),
          ncol=4,
          dimnames=list(names(isomer.conf.par$psi),
            c("parameters","std","lower bound","upper bound" ))))
```

(Results are shown Table 2.3, page 44.)

Confidence Regions for Parameters

We use the functions `ellips` and `iso` and the graphical functions of S-Plus to plot confidence ellipsoids and likelihood contours in the space of the parameters (θ_1, θ_2):

```
> isomer.ell <- ellips(isomer.nl1, axis=c(1,2))
> isomer.cont <- iso(isomer.nl1, axis=c(1,2),
            bounds=matrix(c(25,50,0.03,0.11),nrow=2))
>     # Graphical functions of Splus
> par(mfrow=c(1,2))
> contour(isomer.ell,levels=qchisq(c(0.90,0.95,0.99),4),labex=0)
> points(x=isomer.nl1$theta[1], y=isomer.nl1$theta[2])
> title("Confidence ellipses")
> contour(isomer.cont,levels=qchisq(c(0.90,0.95,0.99),4),labex=0)
> title("Likelihood contours")
> points(x=isomer.nl1$theta[1], y=isomer.nl1$theta[2])
```

(See Figure 2.4, page 45.)

Calculation of Confidence Intervals Using Bootstrap

Confidence intervals using the bootstrap method (see Section 2.3.5, page 35) are calculated using the function `bootstrap`.

Here, to reduce the execution time, which may be long because the model must be calculated several times at each loop, we choose to evaluate by the C program rather than by syntaxical trees (see the Ovocytes Example, Section 1.6, page 24).

To generate the program that calculates the model, we type the operating system command:

```
$ analDer isomer.mod1
```

We then load the program into our S-Plus session:

```
> loadnls2("isomer.mod1.c")
```

To initialize the iterative bootstrap process, **nls2** is first called with the option **renls2**, and, finally, the function **delnls2** cleans the internal structures:

```
> isomer.nl1 <- nls2(isomer,"isomer.mod1", c(36,.07,.04,.2),
          control=list(freq=0), renls2=T)
> isomer.boot <- bootstrap(isomer.nl1,
          method="residuals", n.loops=199)
> delnls2()
```

Histograms of $(\widehat{T}^{\star,b}, b = 1, \dots 199)$ for Each Parameter

Histograms of $\widehat{T}^\star$ for each parameter illustrate the boostrap estimation of their distribution. Only the results corresponding to correct estimations, i.e., when isomer.boot$code=0, are taken into account:

```
> pStar_ isomer.boot$pStar[isomer.boot$code==0,]
> var.pStar_ isomer.boot$var.pStar[isomer.boot$code==0,]
> theta<-matrix(rep(isomer.nl1$theta,isomer.boot$n.loops),
          ncol=4, byrow=T)
> TT <-(pStar - theta)/ sqrt(var.pStar)
> par(mfrow=c(2,2))
> for (a in 1:4)
> {
> hist(TT[,a],probability=T,main="Isomerization example",
    sub=paste("Histogram of bootstrap estimations for T",a),xlab="")
> qx<-seq(from=min(TT[,a]),to=max(TT[,a]),length=75)
> lines(qx,dnorm(qx))
> }
```

(See Figure 2.5, page 46.)

Bootstrap Estimations of Standard Error and Bias for Each Parameter Estimator

We calculate the accuracy characteristics of the bootstrap estimation and display the values of the standard error ($\widehat{S}^\star$), the bias ($\widehat{BIAS}^\star$), the percentage of bias, the 0.0025 and 0.975 percentiles ($b_{0.025}$ and $b_{0.975}$), and the confidence interval $\widehat{I}_B$:

```
> SE.boot <- sqrt(diag(var(pStar)))
> bias.boot <-  apply(pStar,2,mean)-isomer.nl1$theta
> Pbias.boot <- 100*bias.boot/isomer.nl1$theta
> b0.025.boot <- apply(TT,2,quantile,probs=0.025)
```

```
> b0.975.boot <- apply(TT,2,quantile,probs=0.975)
> binf.boot <- isomer.nl1$theta -
          b0.975.boot*coef(isomer.nl1)$std.error
> bsup.boot <- isomer.nl1$theta -
          b0.025.boot*coef(isomer.nl1)$std.error
>    # Print the results:
> print(matrix(c(SE.boot, bias.boot,Pbias.boot,
                 b0.025.boot,b0.975.boot,
                 binf.boot, bsup.boot), ncol=7,
        dimnames=list(names(isomer.nl1$theta),
            c("S","BIAS","% of BIAS","b0.025","b0.975",
              "lower bound","upper bound" ))))
```

Note: The bootstrap method generates different numbers on each execution. Thus, results of these commands may vary slightly from those displayed in Section 2.4, page 46.

Confidence Intervals Using a New Parameterization of the Function f

A new parameterization of the regression function f is considered. The model of Equation (2.10), page 47, is defined in a file called isomer.mod2:

```
resp r;
varind H,P,I;
aux a1, a2;
parresp b1,b2,b3,b4;
subroutine;
begin
a1= P - I/1.632;
a2= b1 + b2*H + b3*P + b4*I;
r=a1/a2;
end
```

Before calling nls2 to estimate the parameters, we have to call the function loadnls2. If we do not do this, the program isomer.mod1.c, previously loaded into the S-Plus session, will still be current. loadnls2 is called without any argument to reset the default action; the default is to calculate the model by syntaxical trees:

```
> loadnls2(psi="")
>  isomer.nl2<-nls2(isomer,"isomer.mod2",rep(1,4))
```

Confidence intervals are calculated using the function confidence.
We display the estimated values of the parameters, their standard errors $(\widehat{S})$, and the 95% confidence interval $\widehat{I}_N$:

```
> isomer.conf.par2 <- confidence(isomer.nl2)
> print(matrix(c(isomer.conf.par2$psi,
                 isomer.conf.par2$std.error,
                 isomer.conf.par2$normal.conf.int[,"lower"],
```

```
           isomer.conf.par2$normal.conf.int[,"upper"]),
     ncol=4,
     dimnames=list(names(isomer.conf.par2$psi),
            c("parameters","S",
              "lower bound","upper bound" ))))
```

(Results are given in Table 2.5, page 47.)

Confidence Regions with the New Parameterization

We plot confidence ellipses and likelihood contours in the space of the parameters (β_1, β_2) using the functions ellips and iso and graphical functions of S-Plus:

```
> isomer.ell2 <- ellips(isomer.nl2, axis=c(1,2))
> isomer.iso2 <- iso(isomer.nl2, axis=c(1,2))
>    # Graphical functions of Splus
> par(mfrow=c(1,2))
> plot(x=c(-5,7),y=c(0.03,.07),type="n",xlab="b1",ylab="b2")
> contour(isomer.ell2,levels=qchisq(c(0.90,0.95,0.99),4),
          add=T,labex=0)
> points(x=isomer.nl2$theta[1], y=isomer.nl2$theta[2])
> title("Confidence ellipses")
> plot(x=c(-5,7),y=c(0.03,.07),type="n",xlab="b1",ylab="b2")
> contour(isomer.iso2,levels=qchisq(c(0.90,0.95,0.99),4),
          add=T,labex=0)
> title("Likelihood contours")
```

(See Figure 2.6, page 48.)

Pasture Regrowth Example: Confidence Interval for $\lambda = \exp\theta_3$

Let us return to the pasture regrowth example to calculate a confidence interval for $\lambda = \exp\theta_3$.

We define the function λ in a file called **pasture.lambda**:

```
psi lambda;
ppsi p3;
subroutine;
begin
lambda = exp(p3);
end
```

A confidence interval for λ is calculated using the confidence function. We display the values of $\widehat{\lambda}$, $\widehat{S}$, $\nu_{0.975}$, and $\widehat{I}_{\mathcal{N}}$:

```
> loadnls2(psi="")
> pasture.conf.expP3 <- confidence(pasture.nl1,
            file="pasture.lambda")
```

```
>    # Print the results:
> cat("Estimated value of lambda:", pasture.conf.expP3$psi,"\n" )
> cat("Estimated value of S:",pasture.conf.expP3$std.error,"\n" )
> cat("nu_(0.975):", qnorm(0.975),"\n" )
> cat("Estimated value of In for exp(p3):",
     pasture.conf.expP3$normal.conf.int,"\n" )
> cat("Estimated value of In for p3:",
     pasture.conf.par$normal.conf.int[3,],"\n" )
> cat("Exponential transformation of the preceding interval:",
     exp(pasture.conf.par$normal.conf.int[3,]),"\n" )
```

(Results for this example are given in Section 2.4.6, page 47.)

3
Variance Estimation

In the radioimmunological assay of cortisol example, we introduced the necessity of using nonlinear regression models with heterogeneous variances, and we suggested the weighted least squares method for analyzing this particular data set (see Sections 1.1.2, 1.3, and 2.4.2). This method, however, is not adequate for every situation. Whereas the radioimmunological assay of cortisol data provided many replications for each variance, some data sets only provide a few replications, and some provide none at all, as we will illustrate in the examples herein.

Although one can feasibly use the weighted least squares method for few replications, it is not the best option because the accuracy of the empirical variance as an estimator of the true variance is rather bad: With four replications, the relative error is roughly 80%. The weighting by such inaccurate estimators can be very misleading.

To handle these situations with few or no replications and to still account for the heterogeneity of the variances, we present three alternative methods in this chapter: The maximum likelihood, the quasi-likelihood, and the three-step methods. All of these are based on a parametric modeling of the variance.

Other methods are also available to solve the estimation problem for *nonlinear heteroscedastic regressions*. For example, R.J. Carroll and D. Ruppert [CR88] propose to take into account heteroscedasticity and skewness by transforming both the data and the regression function, and S.L. Beal and L.B. Sheiner [BS88] describe and compare several estimation methods for dealing with these models.

3.1 Examples

3.1.1 Growth of Winter Wheat Tillers: Few Replications

In [FM88], Faivre and Masle consider the growth of winter wheat, focusing on the differences in the dry weights of the wheat tillers, or stems. Time is

measured on a cumulative degree-days scale with a 0°C base temperature and
a point of origin determined by the physiological state of the plants. Plants
growing on randomly chosen small areas of about 0.15 m^2 are harvested each
week. Table 3.1 and Figure 3.1 document the tiller data, listing the means of
the dry weights of the tillers for plants harvested from the same area.

Table 3.1. Data for the growth of winter wheat tillers

Sum of Degree-Days (base 0°C)	Dry Matter Weight (mg)			
405.65	113.386	90.500		
498.75	161.600	207.650		
567.25	309.514	246.743		
618.30	460.686	422.936		
681.45	1047.000	972.383	1072.022	1034.000
681.45	1169.767	1141.883	999.633	1266.290
681.45	868.662	1133.287		

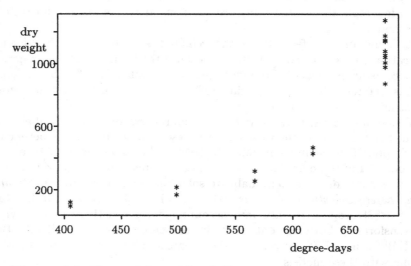

Figure 3.1. Observed dry weight of tillers on a degree-days time scale

The regression equation chosen to describe the increase in dry matter
with respect to the cumulative sum of temperatures is the simple exponential
function

$$f(x, \theta) = \theta_1 \exp(\theta_2 x). \tag{3.1}$$

Here, θ_2 is simply the relative growth rate. As $\exp(0) = 1$, θ_1 could be interpreted as the dry weight of the tillers at the origin; however, a precise physiological interpretation of θ_1 on this basis is risky.

Even though the design of the experiment is highly unbalanced, the variation of the variance of the dry weight with respect to the cumulative sum of temperatures is obvious. Figure 3.2 shows that the intra-replications variances vary with respect to the mean of the observations made at the same time.

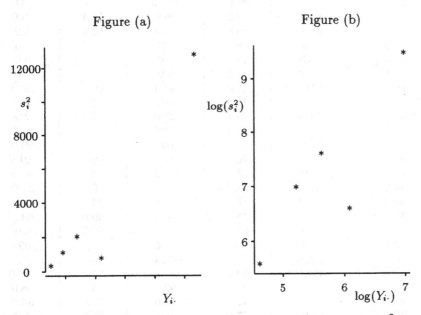

Figure 3.2. Winter wheat tillers example: (a) the empirical variances, s_i^2, versus the mean for the tillers data $Y_i.$; (b) the same data after the logarithm transformation

Although the relative position of the data point corresponding to the fourth harvesting date is troublesome, we can represent the variance of the observations by an increasing function of the response function, $\sigma_i^2 = \sigma^2 f(x_i, \theta)$, for example.

3.1.2 Solubility of Peptides in Trichloacetic Acid Solutions: No Replications

In [CY92], Chabanet and Yvon describe an experiment designed to investigate the precipitation mechanism of peptides. The percentage of solubility of 75 peptides, issued from the digestion of caseins, is related to their retention time on a column of a reverse-phase high-performance liquid chromatography device. The experiment is performed for various trichloacetic acid concentrations; in Table 3.2 and Figure 3.3 we present the data, henceforth called the peptide data, for only one of these concentrations.

Table 3.2. RP-HPLC retention time and solubility of 75 peptides

Retention Time	% Solubility	Ret. Time	% Solubility	Ret. Time	% Solubility
3.6	100.0	3.6	100.0	6.7	99.0
11.2	105.0	20.0	100.0	21.5	84.0
24.5	100.0	29.2	99.0	38.4	88.0
40.4	48.0	49.8	35.0	59.6	0.0
64.2	0.0	68.1	0.0	72.7	0.0
40.8	50.0	52.7	2.0	57.7	0.0
59.1	0.0	61.7	0.0	65.7	0.0
28.3	104.0	33.0	89.0	40.0	56.0
44.5	10.0	47.0	0.0	63.1	0.0
31.6	91.0	40.1	32.0	52.4	2.0
57.5	4.0	23.8	100.0	29.1	85.0
30.0	95.0	31.7	100.0	23.1	95.0
42.7	85.0	46.8	95.0	16.8	101.0
24.0	100.0	31.1	107.0	32.3	84.0
34.0	92.0	34.7	94.0	36.3	97.0
39.3	95.0	42.0	0.0	44.4	51.0
45.0	0.0	46.2	70.0	49.0	63.0
52.1	1.0	55.4	0.0	56.7	0.0
53.0	0.0	0.0	82.0	3.1	102.0
4.2	100.0	7.1	100.0	9.0	95.0
10.6	106.0	13.0	93.0	14.2	107.0
15.5	98.0	38.3	92.0	43.5	48.0
45.9	90.0	47.5	65.0	48.9	34.0
55.6	8.0	57.0	0.0	59.2	1.0
60.9	0.0	34.3	100.0	51.5	0.0

The graph of the data presents the classical S shape, making the logistic function the natural candidate for the regression model. Moreover, as percentages are considered, the asymptotes are, respectively, 0 and 100. Further, it seems likely that these data have heterogeneous variances. No replications are available to obtain estimates of the variance function for each value of the independent variable; however, that the data are percentages suggests some binomial sampling scheme behind the observed phenomena. Hence, we can use a parabola to model the variance: When the peptide is fully nonsoluble, its solubility can be assessed with great precision, while the variability of the measure is maximum for intermediate solubilities. The proposed model is as follows:

$$f(x, \theta) = \frac{100}{1 + \exp\left(\theta_2 \left(x - \theta_1\right)\right)} \tag{3.2}$$

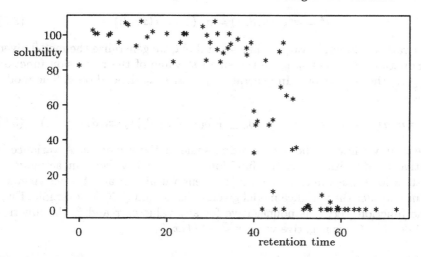

Figure 3.3. Peptides example: Observed solubility of 75 peptides versus their RP-HPLC retention time

and
$$\sigma_i^2 = \sigma^2 + \sigma^2 \tau f(x_i, \theta) \left[100 - f(x_i, \theta)\right] = \sigma^2 g\left(x_i, \theta, \tau\right). \tag{3.3}$$

When x varies from 0 to $+\infty$, $f(x, \theta)$ decreases from 100 to 0, whereas $\sigma^2 g\left(x_i, \theta, \tau\right)$ equals σ^2 when $f(x_i, \theta)$ equals 0, then increases and decreases and has a finite maximal value.

Actually, looking carefully at the data, it appears that the variability is greater when the peptide is fully soluble than when it is nonsoluble. This behavior is not taken into account by the preceding variance function, but this example will be discussed again in Chapter 4.

3.2 Parametric Modeling of the Variance

Before we can estimate the variances, we must choose a variance function. In some cases, this choice can be made on a more or less theoretical basis. But more often, we have only qualitative indications: Either the variance of the observations grows with their expectation, or the relation between the variance of the observations and their expectation can be depicted by a parabola, for example. In both cases, the choice of the model is based on the residuals inside a restricted collection of possible models.

For an increasing variance, there are essentially two models. Either the variance varies as a power of the response

$$\sigma_i^2 = \sigma^2 g\left(x_i, \theta, \tau\right) = \sigma^2 f(x_i, \theta)^\tau, \tag{3.4}$$

or the variance varies as a linear function of the response

$$\sigma_i^2 = \sigma^2 g\left(x_i, \theta, \tau\right) = \sigma^2 \left(1 + \tau f(x_i, \theta)\right). \tag{3.5}$$

For a variance function varying like a parabola, we generalize the model given by Equation (3.3). Let $y_{\min}$ be the smallest value of the regression function and $y_{\max}$ the biggest one. In general, $y_{\min}$ and $y_{\max}$ depend on θ. The model is then

$$\sigma_i^2 = \sigma^2 g\left(x_i, \theta, \tau\right) = \sigma^2 + \sigma^2 \tau_1 \left(y_{\max} + \tau_2 - f(x_i, \theta)\right)\left(f(x_i, \theta) - y_{\min}\right). \tag{3.6}$$

Note that we have to be careful using some of these models. A variance is positive by definition, but the functions mentioned earlier can actually be negative for some values of the independent variable x and the parameters. Let us consider the variance model given by Equation (3.5) for example. Even if the function $f(x, \theta)$ is nonnegative for any value of x and θ, the function $\sigma^2 \left(1 + \tau f(x, \theta)\right)$ is negative when $\tau < -1/f(x, \theta)$.

3.3 Estimation

3.3.1 Maximum Likelihood Estimation

The maximum likelihood method is widely known and is used in the field of parametric inference. Statisticians like it because it behaves well in both theory and practice.

Consider the nonlinear regression model

$$\left. \begin{array}{c} Y_i = f(x_i, \theta) + \varepsilon_i, \\ \mathrm{Var}(\varepsilon_i) = \sigma^2 g\left(x_i, \theta, \tau\right), \ \mathrm{E}(\varepsilon_i) = 0 \end{array} \right\}, \tag{3.7}$$

where the ε_i are assumed to be independent Gaussian random variables for i varying from 1 to n. Note that the parameters θ may enter both the regression and variance functions, while the parameters τ enter the variance function only.

For ease of handling, we generally use the logarithm of the likelihood (log-likelihood for short) instead of the likelihood itself. For the preceding heteroscedastic regression model, the log-likelihood is defined as follows:

$$V(\theta, \sigma^2, \tau) = -\frac{n}{2}\log 2\pi - \frac{1}{2}\sum_{i=1}^{n}\left[\log \sigma^2 g\left(x_i, \theta, \tau\right) + \frac{(Y_i - f(x_i, \theta))^2}{\sigma^2 g\left(x_i, \theta, \tau\right)}\right]. \tag{3.8}$$

For a given set of observations $Y_1, \ldots, Y_n$, the log-likelihood is a function of the parameters. If p is the dimension of θ and q is the dimension of τ, the model depends on $p + q + 1$ parameters. The maximum likelihood estimator $\widehat{\theta}, \widehat{\sigma}^2, \widehat{\tau}$ maximizes the log-likelihood. The values of $\widehat{\theta}, \widehat{\sigma}^2, \widehat{\tau}$ cannot be given explicitly; they are obtained by numerical computation.

Following the calculations done in Section 1.3, let us show how the likelihood is calculated. We observe n independent Gaussian variables $Y_i, i = 1, \ldots n$ with expectation

$\mathrm{E}(Y_i) = f(x_i, \theta)$ and variance $\mathrm{Var}(Y_i) = \sigma^2 g(x_i, \theta, \tau)$. The probability density of the observations calculated in $y_i, i = 1, \ldots n$, is equal to $\prod_{i=1}^{n} \ell(y_i, x_i, \theta, \sigma^2, \tau)$, where the function ℓ is defined as follows:

$$\ell(y, x, \theta, \sigma^2, \tau) = \frac{1}{\sqrt{2\pi\sigma^2 g(x, \theta, \tau)}} \exp\left(-\frac{(y - f(x, \theta))^2}{2\sigma^2 g(x, \theta, \tau)}\right).$$

The likelihood function is thus defined by the following formula:

$$L(Y_1, \ldots, Y_n; \theta, \sigma^2, \tau) = \prod_{i=1}^{n} \ell(Y_i, x_i, \theta, \sigma^2, \tau).$$

3.3.2 Quasi-Likelihood Estimation

The maximum likelihood estimator defined earlier is based on the assumption that the errors ε_i for i varying from 1 to n are distributed as Gaussian variables. In some cases this assumption is not appropriate. For example, when we observe counts or proportions, it is more appropriate to model the distribution of the errors ε_i with a Poisson or binomial distribution. Such data will be considered in Chapters 6 and 7. In other situations we would satisfy ourselves by considering the nonlinear regression (3.7) without any additional assumption on the error distribution. For estimating the parameters, we can use the quasi-likelihood method based on the knowledge of the regression and variance functions only. We will distinguish two cases according to the parametric modeling of the variance function. More precisely, we first consider the case where the parameter τ is known and then the case where the parameter τ is unknown and has to be estimated.

When the Parameter τ is Known We assume that the variance of ε_i is proportional to a known function g that depends on the independent variable x_i and on the unknown parameters θ. For example, consider the variance function defined in Equation (3.4) with $\tau = 2$. More generally we consider the nonlinear regression model

$$\left.\begin{array}{c} Y_i = f(x_i, \theta) + \varepsilon_i, \\ \mathrm{Var}(\varepsilon_i) = \sigma^2 g(x_i, \theta), \ \mathrm{E}(\varepsilon_i) = 0 \end{array}\right\}, \tag{3.9}$$

where the ε_i are assumed to be independent random variables for i varying from 1 to n.

The quasi-likelihood equations are given by the formulas

$$U_a(\theta) = \sum_{i=1}^{n} \frac{\partial f}{\partial \theta_a}(x_i, \theta) \frac{Y_i - f(x_i, \theta)}{g(x_i, \theta)}, \text{ for } a = 1, \ldots, p, \tag{3.10}$$

where for each $a = 1, \ldots, p$,

$$\frac{\partial f}{\partial \theta_a}(x_i, \theta)$$

denotes the derivative of f with respect to θ_a calculated in x_i and θ.

The quasi-likelihood estimators of θ and σ^2 denoted by $\widehat{\theta}_{QL}$ and $\widehat{\sigma}^2_{QL}$, are defined as follows:

$$U_a(\widehat{\theta}_{QL}) = 0 \text{ for } a = 1, \ldots, p$$

and

$$\widehat{\sigma}^2_{QL} = \frac{1}{n} \sum_{i=1}^{n} \frac{(Y_i - f(x_i, \widehat{\theta}_{QL}))^2}{g(x_i, \widehat{\theta}_{QL})}.$$

Note that if the variance of the observations is constant $(g(x, \theta, \tau) = 1)$, the quasi-likelihood estimator and the least squares estimator are the same; see Equation (1.12).

When the Parameter τ is Unknown Let us come back to the nonlinear regression model given by Equation (3.7). We have to estimate θ with p components, τ with q components, and σ^2. The quasi-likelihood equations are given by the formulas

$$U_a(\theta, \tau) = \sum_{i=1}^{n} \frac{\partial f}{\partial \theta_a}(x_i, \theta) \frac{Y_i - f(x_i, \theta)}{g(x_i, \theta, \tau)}, \text{ for } a = 1, \ldots, p, \quad (3.11)$$

$$U_{p+b}(\theta, \tau) = \sum_{i=1}^{n} \frac{\partial g}{\partial \tau_b}(x_i, \theta, \tau) \frac{(Y_i - f(x_i, \theta))^2 - \sigma^2 g(x_i, \theta, \tau)}{g^2(x_i, \theta, \tau)}, \quad (3.12)$$

for b = 1, ..., q. The quasi-likelihood estimators $\widehat{\theta}_{QL}$, $\widehat{\tau}_{QL}$, and $\widehat{\sigma}^2_{QL}$ satisfy

$$\left.\begin{array}{l} U_a(\widehat{\theta}_{QL}, \widehat{\tau}_{QL}) = 0 \text{ for } a = 1, \ldots, p, \\ U_{p+b}(\widehat{\theta}_{QL}, \widehat{\tau}_{QL}) = 0 \text{ for } b = 1, \ldots, q, \end{array}\right\} \quad (3.13)$$

and

$$\widehat{\sigma}^2_{QL} = \frac{1}{n} \sum_{i=1}^{n} \frac{(Y_i - f(x_i, \widehat{\theta}_{QL}))^2}{g(x_i, \widehat{\theta}_{QL}, \widehat{\tau}_{QL})}.$$

Let us comment on the choice of the weighting function in the quasi-likelihood equations. For the first p Equations (3.11), the weighting function is simply the variance function. For the last q equations, we choose the weighting function as the square of the variance function. This choice is based on the following remark: The variance of ε^2, where ε is a centered Gaussian random variable with variance σ^2, equals $2\sigma^4$. The quasi-likelihood equations are defined as if the moments of order 4 of the variables ε_i, say $E(\varepsilon_i^4)$, were equal to the moments of centered Gaussian variables.

We will compare the maximum likelihood method with the quasi-likelihood method in Section 3.5.2. Note that if the ε_i are independent Gaussian variables for i varying from 1 to n, then the quasi-likelihood estimator and the maximum likelihood estimator are not the same. Based on our own experience and the research, we strongly encourage the user to adopt the maximum likelihood approach if there is no particular reason to question the Gaussian assumption.

3.3.3 Three-Step Estimation

For some cases, such as the model in Equation (3.7), the number of parameters is large, making the direct numerical maximization of the log-likelihood with respect to the complete set of parameters or the resolution of the set of Equations (3.13) difficult. To overcome this difficulty, we can use the *three-step method*. This method breaks down the estimation process into successive easier-to-handle steps, as we describe when we estimate the parameters by the quasi-likelihood method.

Step 1: Ordinary Least Squares Estimation of θ A first estimator of θ is $\widehat{\theta}_{OLS(1)}$, which minimizes $C(\theta) = \sum_{i=1}^{n} (Y_i - f(x_i, \theta))^2$ (see Section 1.3).

Step 2: Estimation of τ by the Quasi-Likelihood Method The value of the parameter θ is assumed to be known and is given by its estimation from the preceding step, say $\widehat{\theta}_{OLS(1)}$. Then we estimate τ using the quasi-likelihood method: $\widehat{\tau}_{QL(2)}$ satisfies $U_{p+b}(\widehat{\theta}_{OLS(1)}, \widehat{\tau}_{QL(2)}) = 0$ for $b = 1, \ldots, q$.

Step 3: Estimation of θ by the Quasi-Likelihood Method Finally, we estimate θ and σ^2 using the quasi-likelihood method, assuming that the value of τ is known and equals $\widehat{\tau}_{QL(2)}$. More exactly, the estimator $\widehat{\theta}_{QL(3)}$ is defined by $U_a(\widehat{\theta}_{QL(3)}, \widehat{\tau}_{QL(2)}) = 0$ for $a = 1, \ldots, p$ and

$$\sigma^2_{QL(3)} = \frac{1}{n} \sum_{i=1}^{n} \frac{(Y_i - f(x_i, \widehat{\theta}_{QL(3)}))^2}{g(x_i, \widehat{\theta}_{QL(3)}, \widehat{\tau}_{QL(2)})}.$$

This three-step estimation method has good properties: We can obtain classical asymptotic results analogous to the ones described in Section 2.3.1. Moreover, it is of particular interest if the user is faced with numerical difficulties, as can happen if reasonable initial values of the parameters are not easy to find.

In the second and third steps of the three-step alternative method, the maximum likelihood method can be used in place of the quasi-likelihood method.

3.4 Tests and Confidence Regions

3.4.1 The Wald Test

Each of the methods described in the preceding section has good properties: We can obtain classical asymptotic results analogous to the ones described in Section 2.3.1. As a consequence, for a continuous real function of the parameters $\lambda(\theta, \sigma^2, \tau)$, we have the following results. Let $\widehat{\theta}, \widehat{\sigma}^2, \widehat{\tau}$ be the estimates of θ, σ^2, τ obtained by either of the methods that we considered in the preceding section. Denote $\widehat{\lambda} = \lambda(\widehat{\theta}, \widehat{\sigma}^2, \widehat{\tau})$ and $\lambda = \lambda(\theta, \sigma^2, \tau)$. Then $\widehat{\lambda} - \lambda$ tends to 0 as n

tends to infinity. Moreover, there exists an asymptotic estimate $\widehat{S}$ of the standard error of $\widehat{\lambda}$ such that the distribution of $\widehat{S}^{-1}(\widehat{\lambda} - \lambda)$ can be approximated by a standard Gaussian distribution $\mathcal{N}(0, 1)$. As in Section 2.3.3, we can test hypothesis H: $\{\lambda = \lambda_0\}$, against the alternative A: $\{\lambda \neq \lambda_0\}$, using the Wald statistic

$$\mathcal{S}_{\mathrm{W}} = \frac{(\widehat{\lambda} - \lambda_0)^2}{\widehat{S}^2}.$$

To this end, we use the following decision rule. We choose a risk level α, $\alpha < 1$; then we compute the critical value C such that $\Pr\{Z_1 > C\} = \alpha$, where Z_1 is a random variable distributed as a χ^2 with one degree of freedom; then we compare $\mathcal{S}_{\mathrm{W}}$ and C: If $\mathcal{S}_{\mathrm{W}} > C$, we reject hypothesis H; if $\mathcal{S}_{\mathrm{W}} \leq C$, we do not reject it. This test has an asymptotic level α.

Remarks

1. We have already seen various examples for λ in a homoscedastic regression model in Section 2.4. So we can easily imagine what type of function of the parameters we can consider for inference in a heteroscedastic model, taking into account that the variance parameters (σ^2 and τ) also may appear in such a function. A very simple example is provided by $\lambda = \tau$ in the model given by Equation (3.3) when analyzing the peptide data.
2. We have presented the Wald test without distinguishing among the maximum likelihood method, the quasi-likelihood method, and the three-step method because the computations are formally the same. Obviously, because all the methods are based on the fulfillment of distinct criteria, they do not give the same numerical results for a given set of observations. See Section 3.5.2 for an illustration.
3. We have developed the Wald test only for a real (scalar) function of the parameters. This can be extended to r-dimensional functions of the parameters as in Section 2.3.4, where r is not greater than the total number of parameters.

3.4.2 The Likelihood Ratio Test

In Section 2.3.3, the likelihood ratio test statistic $\mathcal{S}_{\mathrm{L}}$ was introduced for a regression model with homogeneous variances, where the estimation method is ordinary least squares. In that case, the computation of the statistic $\mathcal{S}_{\mathrm{L}}$ was a particular case application of the general inference methodology based on the maximum likelihood principle. In this section, we describe how this principle applies when we are faced with a heteroscedastic regression model.

In order to treat this point with some generality, let us introduce some notation. We call ϕ the whole set of parameters $\phi^T = (\theta^T \sigma^2 \tau^T)$. We call q the dimension of τ, so ϕ is of dimension $p + q + 1$. For example, in the model described by Equations (3.2) and (3.3) for the peptide data, $p = 2$, $q = 1$, and $\phi = (\theta_1, \theta_2, \sigma^2, \tau)^T$ is a four-dimensional vector. In a lot of situations, $q = 0$, for example, if we describe the variance by $\sigma_i^2 = \sigma^2 f(x_i, \theta)$ as for the tiller data or by $\sigma_i^2 = \sigma^2 f(x_i, \theta)^2$ as for the cortisol data.

We now consider a rather general situation where hypothesis H is described by a linear constraint on a subset of the whole set of parameters ϕ. The constraint is expressed as $\Lambda\phi = L_0$, where Λ is an $r \times (p + q + 1)$ matrix $(r < p+q+1)$ and L_0 is a constant vector with dimension r. r is also assumed to be the rank of the matrix Λ. Let $\widehat{\phi}_H^T = (\widehat{\theta}_H^T, \widehat{\sigma}_H^2, \widehat{\tau}_H^T)$ be the parameter estimators for hypothesis H, which means that the constraint $\Lambda\widehat{\phi}_H = L_0$ is fulfilled, whereas $\widehat{\theta}, \widehat{\sigma}^2, \widehat{\tau}$, the classical maximum likelihood estimators of the parameters of model (3.7), are the parameter estimators for the unconstrained alternative A. The likelihood ratio statistic is

$$S_L = -2\log \frac{L_n(Y_1, \ldots, Y_n; \widehat{\theta}, \widehat{\sigma}^2, \widehat{\tau})}{L_n(Y_1, \ldots, Y_n; \widehat{\theta}_H, \widehat{\sigma}_H^2, \widehat{\tau}_H)} . \tag{3.14}$$

With our notations, this turns out to be

$$S_L = \sum_{i=1}^n \log \frac{\widehat{\sigma}_H^2 g(x_i, \widehat{\theta}_H, \widehat{\tau}_H)}{\widehat{\sigma}^2 g(x_i, \widehat{\theta}, \widehat{\tau})}.$$

Hypothesis H is rejected if $S_L > C$, where C is defined by

$$\Pr\{Z_r \le C\} = 1 - \alpha.$$

Z_r is distributed as a χ^2 with r degrees of freedom, and α is the (asymptotic) level of the test.

Remarks

1. The intuitive justification of this decision rule is clear. On the one hand, if H is true, then both $\widehat{\theta}_H, \widehat{\sigma}_H^2, \widehat{\tau}_H$ and $\widehat{\theta}, \widehat{\sigma}^2, \widehat{\tau}$ are suitable estimators of the model parameters: When the number of observations is large, they are close to the true value of the parameters. Therefore, they take similar values and the likelihood ratio is close to 1, or equivalently, its logarithm is close to 0. On the other hand, if H is false, then $\widehat{\theta}_H, \widehat{\sigma}_H^2, \widehat{\tau}_H$ do not estimate the true value of the parameters and are expected to have values very different from $\widehat{\theta}, \widehat{\sigma}^2, \widehat{\tau}$; thus S_L has a value other than 0.
2. In Section 2.3.3, the test statistic S_L is given by

$$S_L = n \log C(\widehat{\theta}_H) - n \log C(\widehat{\theta}_A).$$

This is the particular form taken by Equation (3.14) in the homogeneous variance situation. Note that for an unconstrained alternative, $\widehat{\theta}_A = \widehat{\theta}$.

3.4.3 Bootstrap Estimations

Following the same idea as in the case of homogeneous variances, the bootstrap estimation of $\lambda = \lambda(\theta, \sigma^2, \tau)$ is based on estimates $\widehat{\lambda}^\star = \lambda(\widehat{\theta}^\star, \widehat{\sigma}^{\star 2}, \widehat{\tau}^\star)$ calculated from artificial bootstrap samples $(x_i, Y_i^\star), i = 1, \ldots, n$, where

$$Y_i^\star = f(x_i, \widehat{\theta}) + \varepsilon_i^\star.$$

The only work we have to do is to generate the errors $(\varepsilon_i^\star, i = 1, \ldots, n)$, such that their distribution mimics the distribution of the $(\varepsilon_i, i = 1, \ldots, n)$. There are several ways to do that. For example, let $(T_i, i = 1, \ldots, n)$ be an n sample of variables independent of $(Y_1, \ldots, Y_n)$, satisfying $\mathrm{E}(T_i) = 0$, $\mathrm{E}(T_i^2) = 1$, and $\mathrm{E}(T_i^3) = 1$; and let $\widehat{\varepsilon}_i = Y_i - f(x_i, \widehat{\theta})$. Then we take $\varepsilon_i^\star = \widehat{\varepsilon}_i T_i$. This method is called *wild bootstrap*. It is easy to find such variables $(T_i, i = 1, \ldots, n)$. Let us consider, for example, $(Z_1, \ldots, Z_n)$ an n sample of Bernoulli variables with parameter $\mu = (5 + \sqrt{5})/10$. Then

$$T_i = \frac{1 - \sqrt{5}}{2} Z_i + \frac{1 + \sqrt{5}}{2}(1 - Z_i) \tag{3.15}$$

is suitable.

If $(\widehat{\theta}, \widehat{\sigma}^2, \widehat{\tau})$ is the maximum likelihood estimator of (θ, σ^2, τ), then $(\widehat{\theta}^\star, \widehat{\sigma}^{\star 2}, \widehat{\tau}^\star)$ will be the value of (θ, σ^2, τ) that minimizes

$$V^\star(\theta, \sigma^2, \tau) = \log L_n(Y_1^\star, \ldots . Y_n^\star, \theta, \sigma^2, \tau).$$

If $(\widehat{\theta}, \widehat{\sigma}^2, \widehat{\tau})$ is the quasi-likelihood estimator or the three-step estimator of (θ, σ^2, τ) then $(\widehat{\theta}^\star, \widehat{\sigma}^{\star 2}, \widehat{\tau}^\star)$ will be the quasi-likelihood estimator or the three-step estimator of (θ, σ^2, τ) obtained when the artificial observations $(Y_i^\star, i = 1, \ldots, n)$ are used in place of the observations $(Y_i, i = 1, \ldots, n)$.

The bootstrap estimate of λ is $\widehat{\lambda}^\star = \lambda(\widehat{\theta}^\star, \widehat{\sigma}^{\star 2}, \widehat{\tau}^\star)$, and the procedures for calculating a bootstrap confidence interval for λ or estimating the accuracy of $\widehat{\lambda}$ are similar to the procedures described in the case of homogeneous variances (see Section 2.3.5).

The way the $(\varepsilon_i^\star, i = 1, \ldots, n)$ are simulated may look a little mysterious. Actually, it can be shown that the moments of $\varepsilon_i^\star$ up to the order 3 are closed to the moments of ε_i. More precisely, if $\mathrm{E}^\star$ denotes the expectation conditional on the observations $(Y_1, \ldots, Y_n)$, we get

$$\mathrm{E}^\star(\varepsilon_i^\star) = 0$$
$$\mathrm{E}^\star\left[(\varepsilon_i^\star)^2\right] = \widehat{\varepsilon}_i^2$$
$$\mathrm{E}^\star\left[(\varepsilon_i^\star)^3\right] = \widehat{\varepsilon}_i^3.$$

These equations give a formal meaning to what we claimed: *To generate the errors* $(\varepsilon_i^\star, i = 1, \ldots, n)$, *such that their distribution* <u>*mimics*</u> *the distribution of the* $(\varepsilon_i, i = 1, \ldots, n)$. More theoretical background may be found in Wu [Wu86] and Liu [Liu88].

3.4.4 Links Between Testing Procedures and Confidence Region Computations

It is generally possible to compute a confidence region from a test procedure and vice versa to perform a test using a confidence region. For example, going back to Section 2.3, we show how the confidence interval $\widehat{I}_N$ given by

Equation (2.2) and the Wald test relate to each other. Actually, both are applications of the same result: The limiting distribution of $\widehat{T} = (\widehat{\lambda} - \lambda)/\widehat{S}$ is a standard normal distribution $\mathcal{N}(0,1)$.

We can easily build a test procedure for hypothesis H: $\{\lambda = \lambda_0\}$ against the alternative A: $\{\lambda \neq \lambda_0\}$, from the confidence interval $\widehat{I}_\mathcal{N}$. The decision rule is simply to reject H if $\widehat{I}_\mathcal{N}$ does not cover λ_0 and to not reject it if λ_0 is covered by $\widehat{I}_\mathcal{N}$. It is not difficult to see that this test procedure exactly corresponds to the Wald test if we take the same asymptotic level α.

On the other hand, we can construct a confidence region for λ by considering the set of all of the values, say ℓ, of λ such that the Wald test does not reject the hypothesis $\{\lambda = \ell\}$. We define this confidence region $\widehat{I}_W$ as follows:

$$\widehat{I}_W = \left\{\ell : \left(\widehat{\lambda} - \ell\right)^2/\widehat{S}^2 \leq C\right\}.$$

Again, if C is such that $\Pr\{Z_1 \leq C\} = 1 - \alpha$, for Z_1 a χ^2 random variable with one degree of freedom, $\widehat{I}_W$ and $\widehat{I}_\mathcal{N}$ do coincide exactly.[1]

This duality between tests and confidence regions is quite general.

3.4.5 Confidence Regions

Let us consider the peptide data and assume that the heteroscedastic regression model given by Equations (3.2) and (3.3) is suitable. Suppose that we want to compute a confidence interval for the parameter θ_2. This parameter is linked to the maximal (in absolute value) slope of the logistic curve, which is $-25\,\theta_2$. Thus it is representative of the variability of the peptide solubility with respect to the retention time.

Let $\widehat{\theta}_1, \widehat{\theta}_2, \widehat{\sigma}^2, \widehat{\tau}$ be the maximum likelihood estimators of the parameters. Here, $\lambda(\theta, \sigma^2, \tau) = \theta_2$ and $\widehat{\lambda} = \widehat{\theta}_2$. $\widehat{S}$ is given simply by the square root of the second term of the diagonal of the matrix estimating the parameter estimates covariance. A confidence interval for θ_2 based on the asymptotic distribution of $\widehat{\theta}_2$ is then just $\widehat{I}_\mathcal{N}$.

We recommend that you compute a confidence interval for θ_2 using the maximum likelihood approach. This method is analogous to the profiling procedure described in [BW88]. To this end, we make use of the previously mentioned duality between tests and confidence regions. Consider first the test of hypothesis H: $\{\theta_2 = \ell\}$, against A: $\{\theta_2 \neq \ell\}$, for a given real positive value ℓ. According to the notation introduced in Section 3.4.2, hypothesis H is described by the linear constraint

$$(0\ 1\ 0\ 0)\begin{pmatrix}\theta_1 \\ \theta_2 \\ \sigma^2 \\ \tau\end{pmatrix} = \ell.$$

---

[1] Recall that C is such that, for $\alpha < 1/2$, $\sqrt{C}$ is the $1 - \alpha/2$ percentile of a standard Gaussian $\mathcal{N}(0,1)$ random variable.

Here, $p = 2$, $q = 1$, and $r = 1$. The computation of the constrained estimators $\widehat{\theta}_{1\,H}, \widehat{\theta}_{2\,H}, \widehat{\sigma}^2_H, \widehat{\tau}_H$ is particularly simple in this case. We consider that θ_2 is no longer an unknown parameter, but a known constant equal to ℓ, and we maximize the likelihood with respect to θ_1, σ^2, τ. To emphasize the dependency on the value ℓ, we adopt another notation, writing $\theta_{1\,\ell}, \sigma^2_\ell, \tau_\ell$ for the estimators obtained under the constraint $\theta_2 = \ell$. With this notation,

$$\mathcal{S}_L = -2\log \frac{L_n(Y_1, \ldots, Y_n; \widehat{\theta}_1, \widehat{\theta}_2, \widehat{\sigma}^2, \widehat{\tau})}{L_n(Y_1, \ldots, Y_n; \widehat{\theta}_{1\,\ell}, \ell, \widehat{\sigma}^2_\ell, \widehat{\tau}_\ell)} \, ,$$

and the decision rule is to reject H if $\mathcal{S}_L > C$, with C given by

$$\Pr\{Z_1 > C\} = \alpha$$

and Z_1 being distributed as a χ^2 with one degree of freedom. We now deduce a confidence region from this test procedure. Obviously, $\mathcal{S}_L$ depends on ℓ and we denote by $\mathcal{S}_L(\ell)$ the value taken by $\mathcal{S}_L$ for a given ℓ. We can define as a confidence region for θ_2 the set of all of the real ℓ such that $\mathcal{S}_L(\ell) \leq C$. In other words, we consider as a confidence region for θ_2 with asymptotic confidence level $1 - \alpha$ the set of all of the real values ℓ such that we do not reject hypothesis H: $\{\theta_2 = \ell\}$, using a likelihood ratio test with asymptotic level α.

Remarks

1. The confidence region $\{\ell : \mathcal{S}_L(\ell) \leq C\}$ cannot be translated into a more explicit form. We use some numerical computations to obtain its endpoints.
2. This type of confidence region based on the log-likelihood ratio can easily be generalized to any subset of the parameter vector ϕ or to any linear function of the type $\Lambda\phi = L_0$, with Λ an $r \times p + q + 1$ matrix of rank r, $r < p + q + 1$, and L_0 an r-dimensional vector.

3.5 Applications

3.5.1 Growth of Winter Wheat Tillers

Model The regression function is

$$f(x, \theta) = \theta_1 \exp(\theta_2 x),$$

and the variance function is $\mathrm{Var}(\varepsilon_i) = \sigma^2 f(x_i, \theta)$.

Method The parameters are estimated by maximizing the log-likelihood, $V(\theta, \sigma^2, \tau)$; see Equation (3.8).

Results

Parameters	Estimated Values	Asymptotic Covariance Matrix	
θ_1	1.14	0.24	
θ_2	0.01	-0.0003	4×10^{-7}
σ^2	13.32		

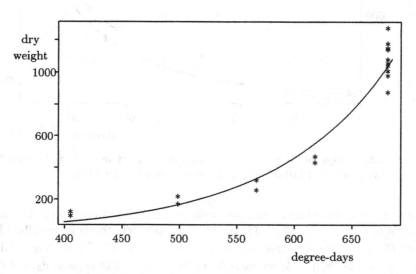

Figure 3.4. Weight of tillers example: Graph of observed and adjusted curve

The adjusted response curve, $f(x, \widehat{\theta})$, is shown in Figure 3.4. A quick inspection of this graph shows that the regression model is not very well chosen. It would be better to have a regression function with a more gradual increase for low values of x. This can be achieved by elevating $\theta_2 x$ to some power, that is, by choosing

$$f(x, \theta) = \theta_1 \exp\left[(\theta_2 x)^{\theta_3}\right], \tag{3.16}$$

where the variance function, as before, is $\mathrm{Var}(\varepsilon_i) = \sigma^2 f(x_i, \theta)$.

Results

Parameters	Estimated Values	Asymptotic Covariance Matrix		
θ_1	79.13	702.2		
θ_2	0.0019	-0.0004	2×10^{-8}	
θ_3	4.05	23.07	10^{-8}	0.85
σ^2	7.30			

Likelihood Ratiof Test of H: $\theta_3 = 1$ against A: $\theta_3 \neq 1$ Using Results of Section 3.4.2 Figure 3.5 suggests that the regression model given by Equation (3.16) fits the tiller data better.

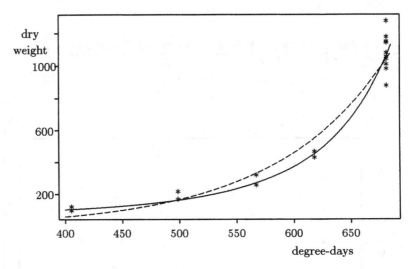

Figure 3.5. Weight of tillers example: Graph of observed and adjusted curves for both the hypothesis H (dashed line) and the alternative A (solid line)

To validate this observation, we perform a likelihood ratio test. The hypothesis to be tested is $\{\theta_3 = 1\}$. In this case, the hypothesis is described by model (3.1), and the alternative is described by model (3.16). So $\widehat{\theta}_{1\,H} = 1.14$, $\widehat{\theta}_{2\,H} = 0.01$, and $\widehat{\theta}_{3\,H} = 1$; whereas $\widehat{\theta}_1 = 79.13$, $\widehat{\theta}_2 = 0.0019$, and $\widehat{\theta}_3 = 4.05$. The statistic S_L is equal to 10.4. If Z_1 is distributed as a χ^2 with one degree of freedom, the critical value C such that $\Pr\{Z_1 \leq C\} = 0.95$ is 3.84. Thus, using the likelihood ratio test with an asymptotic 5% level, we reject hypothesis H.

Calculation of a Confidence Interval for θ_3 Using the Asymptotic Distribution of $\widehat{\theta}_3$ See Section 3.4.5.

$\widehat{\theta}_3$	$\widehat{S}$	$\nu_{0.975}$	$\widehat{I}_{\mathcal{N}}$
4.05	0.924	1.96	[2.239, 5.861]

Calculation of a Confidence Interval for θ_3 Using the Log-Likelihood Ratio See Section 3.4.5.

As mentioned earlier, the computation of a confidence interval based on the log-likelihood ratio requires some extra calculations after we have performed the estimation. Although these calculations are implemented in S-Plus, (see Section 3.6), describing the necessary calculations as follows helps to understand the method better:

1. Choose a *reasonable* set of possible values for θ_3. Here, $\widehat{\theta}_3$ is equal to 4.05, and one estimate of its standard error $\widehat{S}$ is equal to 0.924. We take 39 equispaced values $t_1, t_2, \ldots, t_{39}$ with $t_1 = 1$ and $t_{39} = 7.10$; the central value t_{20} is just $\widehat{\theta}_3$. Note that the choice of this series is quite arbitrary.

We decided to explore the behavior of the log-likelihood ratio for values of θ_3 roughly between $\widehat{\theta}_3 - 3\widehat{S}$ and $\widehat{\theta}_3 + 3\widehat{S}$.

2. For each value t_i, for $i = 1, \ldots, 39$, fix $\theta_3 = t_i$ and estimate the other parameters under this constraint. Then compute the log-likelihood ratio $\mathcal{S}_{\mathrm{L}}(t_i)$ (obviously, $\mathcal{S}_{\mathrm{L}}(t_{20}) = 0$).

3. Draw a picture of $\mathcal{S}_{\mathrm{L}}(\ell)$ versus ℓ. This is a useful step to check the regularity of the log-likelihood and to provide a comprehensive look at the results of the preceding step. On the same graph, draw the horizontal line corresponding to the equation $y = C$. The abscissa of the intersection points between this line and the graph of the log-likelihood are the endpoints of the confidence region based on the log-likelihood ratio.

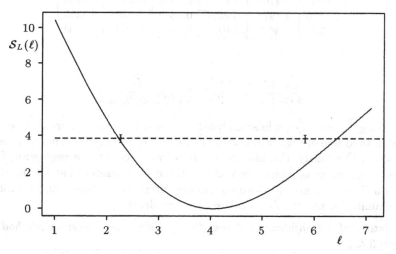

Figure 3.6. Confidence intervals: Values of the log-likelihood ratio when the parameter θ_3 varies ($\theta_3 = \ell$)

4. Determine the endpoints of the confidence region by linear interpolation. Here the picture (see Figure 3.6) clearly shows that the region is an interval. Let us consider the set of values $\mathcal{S}_{\mathrm{L}}(t_i)$, for $i = 1, \ldots, 39$ (see Table 3.3). For a confidence interval with asymptotic level 0.95, choose C such that $\Pr\{Z_1 > C\} = 0.05$, for Z_1 a χ^2 with one degree of freedom: $C = 3.8415$. From Table 3.3, we deduce that the left endpoint of the log-likelihood ratio-based confidence interval is between $t_8 = 2.1237$ and $t_9 = 2.2842$, because $\mathcal{S}_{\mathrm{L}}(t_8) = 4.3269$ and $\mathcal{S}_{\mathrm{L}}(t_9) = 3.6335$. A precise enough value of the lower bound $\widehat{\theta}_{3\,\mathrm{inf}}$ of the confidence interval is given by linear interpolation and is 2.236. Similarly, the right endpoint, or upper bound, $\widehat{\theta}_{3\,\mathrm{sup}}$ of the confidence interval is between t_{34} and t_{35} and is 6.428.

Let us summarize the results of this procedure:

Table 3.3. Log-likelihood values

t	$S_L(t)$	t	$S_L(t)$	t	$S_L(t)$
1.0000	10.4256	3.0868	1.0491	5.1737	1.0856
1.1605	9.4496	3.2474	0.7203	5.3342	1.3781
1.3211	8.5016	3.4079	0.4550	5.4947	1.6940
1.4816	7.5856	3.5684	0.2523	5.6553	2.0302
1.6421	6.7060	3.7289	0.1104	5.8158	2.3835
1.8026	5.8669	3.8895	0.0272	5.9763	2.7513
1.9632	5.0726	4.0500	0.0000	6.1368	3.1308
2.1237	4.3269	4.2105	0.0256	6.2974	3.5198
2.2842	3.6335	4.3711	0.1006	6.4579	3.9162
2.4447	2.9957	4.5316	0.2214	6.6184	4.3180
2.6053	2.4164	4.6921	0.3841	6.7789	4.7236
2.7658	1.8978	4.8526	0.5849	6.9395	5.1315
2.9263	1.4417	5.0132	0.8200	7.1000	5.5403

$\widehat{\theta}_3$	$\widehat{S}$	$\chi^1_{1,0.95}$	$\widehat{I}_S$
4.05	0.924	3.8415	[2.236, 6.428]

Comparing $\widehat{I}_S$ with $\widehat{I}_N$, whose endpoints appear as vertical bars on the horizontal dashed line of Figure 3.6, we observe that $\widehat{I}_S$ is larger and nonsymmetric around $\widehat{\theta}_3$. Obviously, the likelihood takes into account the regression function as it is, whereas using the Wald statistic we consider that the model is almost a linear regression. Both confidence intervals are based on asymptotic approximations, but for $\widehat{I}_N$ this is even more drastic.

Calculation of a Confidence Interval for θ_3 Using the Bootstrap Method See Section 3.4.3.

Table 3.4 gives the estimated values of f, the $\widehat{f}_i$, and the residuals $\widehat{\varepsilon}_i = Y_i - f(x_i, \widehat{\theta})$ for the model defined in Equation (3.16). For two bootstrap simulations, the table gives the values of Z_i, the bootstrap errors $\varepsilon_i^\star$, the bootstrap observations $Y_i^\star$, the bootstrap estimate of θ_3, and the corresponding asymptotic variance $S_{\widehat{\theta}^\star}$.

The number of bootstrap simulations B equals 199. The histogram of the $(\widehat{T}^{\star,b}, b = 1, \ldots, B)$ is shown in Figure 3.7.

The 0.025 and 0.975 percentiles of the $(\widehat{T}^{\star,b}, b = 1, \ldots, B)$ are calculated and then the bootstrap confidence interval is calculated:

$\widehat{\theta}_3$	$\widehat{S}$	$b_{0.025}$	$b_{0.975}$	$\widehat{I}_B$
4.05	0.924	−1.73	1.08	[3.06, 5.65]

3.5.2 Solubility of Peptides in Trichloacetic Acid Solutions

Model The regression function is

Table 3.4. Results for two bootstrap simulations

$\hat{f}_i$	$\tilde{\varepsilon}_i$	Z_i	$\varepsilon_i^{\star,1}$	$Y_i^{\star,1}$	Z_i	$\varepsilon_i^{\star,2}$	$Y_i^{\star,2}$
108.83	4.56	1	-2.80	106.01	1	-2.8	106.01
108.83	-18.30	1	11.00	120.15	1	11.0	120.15
165.16	-3.56	1	2.20	167.37	1	2.2	167.37
165.16	42.50	1	-26.00	138.91	1	-26.0	138.91
273.24	36.30	1	-22.00	250.82	0	59.0	331.93
273.24	-26.50	1	16.00	289.62	1	16.0	289.62
458.50	2.19	1	-1.40	457.15	0	3.5	462.04
458.50	-35.60	1	22.00	480.48	0	-58.0	400.96
1070.60	-23.60	1	15.00	1085.20	1	15.0	1085.20
1070.60	-98.20	1	61.00	1131.30	1	61.0	1131.30
1070.60	1.39	1	-0.86	1069.80	0	2.3	1072.90
1070.60	-36.60	1	23.00	1093.30	1	23.0	1093.30
1070.60	99.10	1	-61.00	1009.40	1	-61.0	1009.40
1070.60	71.30	1	-44.00	1026.60	1	-44.0	1026.60
1070.60	-71.00	0	-110.00	955.76	1	44.0	1114.50
1070.60	196.00	1	-120.00	949.70	1	-120.0	949.70
1070.60	-202.00	0	-330.00	743.84	0	-330.0	743.84
1070.60	62.70	1	-39.00	1031.90	1	-39.0	1031.90
$\hat{\theta}_3 = 4.05, \hat{S} = 0.924$			$\hat{\theta}_3^{\star,1} = 3.73, S_{\hat{\theta}^{\star},1} = 0.874$			$\hat{\theta}_3^{\star,2} = 3.80, S_{\hat{\theta}^{\star},2} = 0.941$	

$$f(x, \theta) = \frac{100}{1 + \exp\left(\theta_2 \left(x - \theta_1\right)\right)},$$

and the variance function is $\mathrm{Var}(\varepsilon_i) = \sigma^2 \left(1 + \tau f(x_i, \theta) \left(100 - f(x_i, \theta)\right)\right)$.

Method The parameters are estimated by maximizing the log-likelihood, $V(\theta, \sigma^2, \tau)$; see Equation (3.8).

Results

Parameters	Estimated Values	Asymptotic Covariance Matrix		
θ_1	43.93	0.3946		
θ_2	0.4332	-1.5×10^{-6}	0.0031	
τ	0.0245	-6.1×10^{-5}	0.0004	8.1×10^{-5}
σ^2	26.79			

The adjusted response curve, $f(x, \hat{\theta})$, is shown in Figure 3.8.

Likelihood Ratio Test of the Existence of a Constant Term in the Variance Model In order to verify that a constant term in the variance is necessary to correctly describe the variability of the data, we perform a test of hypothesis H: $\left\{\mathrm{Var}(\varepsilon_i) = \sigma^2 f(x_i, \theta) \left(100 - f(x_i, \theta)\right)\right\}$. In order to make clear that this is a hypothesis of the type $\Lambda\phi = L_0$, let us rewrite the variance model under A as $\left\{\mathrm{Var}(\varepsilon_i) = \sigma_1^2 + \sigma_2^2 f(x_i, \theta) \left(100 - f(x_i, \theta)\right)\right\}$. In this notation, we express hypothesis H as $\left\{\sigma_1^2 = 0\right\}$. Between this alternative modeling of the variance and the original one given by Equation (3.3), there is only a simple one-to-one

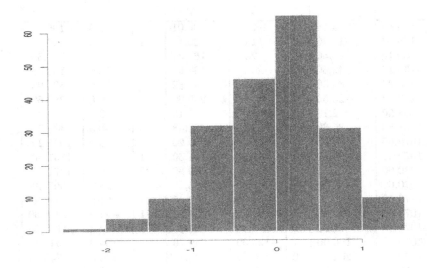

Figure 3.7. Weight of tillers example: Histogram of $(\widehat{T}^{*,b},\, b = 1,\ldots B)$

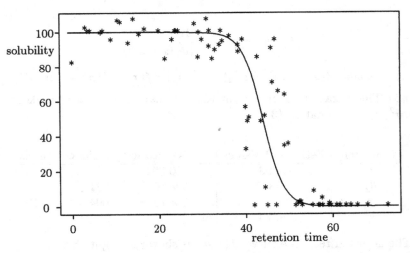

Figure 3.8. Peptides example: Observed and adjusted solubilities of 75 peptides versus their RP-HPLC retention time

transformation: $\sigma_1^2 = \sigma^2$, $\sigma_2^2 = \sigma^2 \tau$. The values of the estimates under this assumption are $\widehat{\theta}_{1\,H} = 41.70$ and $\widehat{\theta}_{2\,H} = 0.1305$. The statistic $\mathcal{S}_L$ is equal to 70.14. Because it is a highly unlikely value for a χ^2 random variable with one degree of freedom, hypothesis H must be rejected.

Figure 3.9 illustrates the observed solubilities, drawn together with the adjusted one under hypothesis H (dashed line) and model (3.2) (solid line). The second line is obviously a better fit.

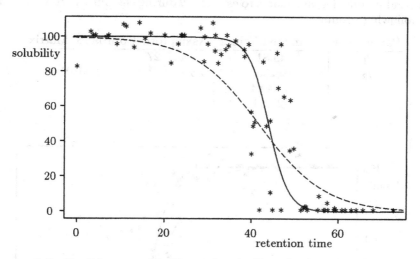

Figure 3.9. Peptides example: Observed and adjusted solubilities of 75 peptides versus their RP-HPLC retention time for both hypothesis H (dashed line) and the alternative A (solid line)

A discerning reader could have foreseen the result of this test. Indeed, assuming that hypothesis H is fulfilled is equivalent to assuming that the extreme measures (corresponding to $f(x, \theta) = 0$ or $f(x, \theta) = 100$) are performed with perfect accuracy. Thus the estimation process gives these extreme measures a very high weight, whereas it barely takes the intermediate data into account. The dashed curve in Figure 3.9, which corresponds to the peptide data fit under hypothesis H, illustrates this fact.

Calculation of a Confidence Interval for θ_2 Using the Log-Likelihood Ratio Using the same type of procedure that we used to compute a confidence interval for θ_3 in Section 3.5.1, we obtain the following result:

$\widehat{\theta}_2$	$\widehat{S}$	$\chi^2_{1,0.95}$	$\widehat{I}_S$
0.433	0.0557	3.8415	[0.309, 0.670]

Calculation of a Confidence Interval for θ_2 Using the Wald Statistic, Based on the Maximum Likelihood Estimator Standard calculations lead to the following result:

$\widehat{\theta}_2$	$\widehat{S}$	$\nu_{0.975}$	$\widehat{I}_{\mathcal{N}}$
0.433	0.0557	1.96	[0.324, 0.542]

Calculation of a Confidence Interval for θ_2 Using the Wald Statistic, Based on the Three-Step Method We introduce, for the sake of comparison, the three-step method for estimating the parameters, using an estimator other than the maximum likelihood estimator. We choose ordinary least squares to estimate θ during the first step, modified least squares to estimate β during the second step, and modified least squares to estimate θ during the third step. We obtain the following results:

Parameters	Estimated Values	Asymptotic Covariance Matrix	
θ_1	43.81	0.7427	
θ_2	0.233	5.8×10^{-4}	0.00101
τ	0.0084		
σ^2	27.56		

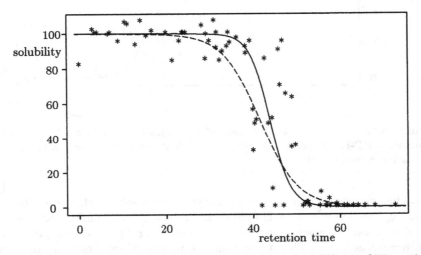

Figure 3.10. Peptides example: Observed and adjusted solubilities of 75 peptides versus their RP-HPLC retention time for both the three-step method (dashed line) and the maximum likelihood method (solid line)

Both estimated regression functions are shown in Figure 3.10.

We can also compute the confidence interval for θ_2 based on the results of this estimation procedure:

$\widehat{\theta}_2$	$\widehat{S}$	$\nu_{0.975}$	$\widehat{I}'_{\mathcal{N}}$
0.233	0.031	1.96	[0.171, 0.295]

Actually, in this example, the results of both estimation methods disagree to a large extent. As far as we trust our modeling of the phenomenon, the three-step method, using modified least squares methods at steps 2 and 3, does not fit the data sufficiently well, as we can see from an examination of Figure 3.10 and by comparing the value of the log-likelihood obtained by both methods: The log-likelihood computed with the values of the three-step estimators is −281.8, whereas the maximum log-likelihood is −288.7. This strongly supports our advice: Use the maximum likelihood method as often as you can!

3.6 Using nls2

This section reproduces the commands and files used in this chapter to treat the examples using **nls2**.

Growth of Winter Wheat Tiller Example

The wheat tiller example is a new example, introduced in this chapter. First we create the *data frame* to store the experimental data. Then we estimate the parameters with two models, and, finally, we calculate confidence intervals to compare them.

Creating the Data

The experimental data (see Table 3.1, page 62) are stored in a *data frame* called `tiller`:

```
> DegreeDays <-c(
  405.65, 405.65, 498.75, 498.75, 567.25, 567.25, 618.30,
  618.30, 681.45, 681.45, 681.45, 681.45, 681.45, 681.45,
  681.45, 681.45, 681.45, 681.45)
> DryWeight <-c(
  113.386,  90.500, 161.600, 207.650, 309.514, 246.743,
  460.686, 422.936, 1047.000, 972.383, 1072.022, 1034.000,
  1169.767, 1141.883, 999.633, 1266.290, 868.662, 1133.287)
> tiller <- data.frame( DegreeDays,  DryWeight)
```

Plot of the Observed Dry Weights on a Degree-Days Time Scale.

We plot the observed response values versus the degree-days scale using the graphical function `plot` of S-Plus:

```
> plot(DegreeDays,DryWeight,xlab="degree days",ylab="dry weight",
    main="Growth of winter wheat tillers example",
    sub="Observed response")
```

(See Figure 3.1, page 62.)

Plot of the Empirical Variance Versus Mean

S-Plus functions are used to calculate empirical intrareplications variances, and means. We plot the empirical variances versus the empirical means and the same plot after the logarithm transformation:

```
> tiller.mean<-as.vector(
      unlist(lapply(split(DryWeight,DegreeDays),mean)))
> tiller.var<-as.vector(
      unlist(lapply(split(DryWeight,DegreeDays),var)))
> plot(tiller.mean, tiller.var, xlab="mean", ylab="var",
      main="Growth of winter wheat tillers example",
      sub="Empirical response variance versus response mean")
> plot(log(tiller.mean), log(tiller.var),
      xlab="log(mean)", ylab="log(var)",
      main="Growth of winter wheat tillers example",
      sub="Log of empirical response variance\
  versus log of response mean")
```

(See Figure 3.2, page 63.)

Parameter Estimation Under Hypothesis H

We describe the model of hypothesis H (the simple exponential function defined in Section 3.5.1, page 74) in a file called `tiller.exp.m2`:

```
% Model simple exponential
%        with response variances proportional
%        to response expectations
resp DryWeight;
varind DegreeDays;
var v;
parresp a,b;
subroutine;
begin
DryWeight= a*exp(b*DegreeDays);
v = DryWeight;
end
```

To find reasonable starting values for the parameters, we make a linear regression of log(dry weight) on degree-days using the function `lm` in S-Plus. Then we call `nls2`. We display the estimated values of the parameters $\hat{\sigma}^2$ and the estimated asymptotic covariance matrix:

```
> tiller.lm <- lm(log(DryWeight) ~ DegreeDays)
> tiller.nl2 <- nls2(tiller,  "tiller.exp.m2",
      c(exp(tiller.lm$coefficients[1]),tiller.lm$coefficients[2]))
>    # Print the results:
> cat( "Estimated values of the parameters:\n ")
> print(tiller.nl2$theta)
```

```
> cat( "\nEstimated value of sigma2:\n ")
> print( tiller.nl2$sigma2)
> cat( "\nEstimated asymptotic covariance matrix: \n ")
> print(tiller.nl2$as.var); cat("\n\n")
```

We plot the observed and fitted response values versus the degree-days scale:

```
> plot(DegreeDays,DryWeight,xlab="degree days",ylab="dry weight",
       main="Growth of winter wheat tillers example",
       sub="Observed response")
> X<-seq(400,685,length=100)
> Y<-tiller.nl2$theta[1]*exp(tiller.nl2$theta[2]*X)
> lines(X,Y)
```

(See Figure 3.4, page 75.)

Parameter Estimation Under Hypothesis A

The second model to test is the double exponential function defined by Equation (3.16), page 75. We describe it in a file called `tiller.exp.m7`:

```
% Model double exponential
%       with response variances proportional
%       to response expectations
resp DryWeight;
varind DegreeDays;
var v;
parresp a,b,g;
subroutine;
begin
DryWeight= a*exp(exp(g*log(DegreeDays*b)));
v = DryWeight;
end
```

The function **nls2** is called to carry out the estimation. The values estimated with the first model are assigned to the starting values of the parameters. Option `max.iters` increases the default maximal number of iterations, so we can be sure that convergence will be reached:

```
> tiller.nl7 <- nls2(tiller, "tiller.exp.m7",
    list(theta.start = c(tiller.nl2$theta, 1), max.iters=500))
>    # Print the results:
> cat( "Estimated values of the parameters:\n ")
> print(tiller.nl7$theta)
> cat( "\nEstimated value of sigma2:\n ")
> print( tiller.nl7$sigma2)
> cat( "\nEstimated asymptotic covariance matrix: \n ")
> print(tiller.nl7$as.var); cat("\n\n")
```

Plots of the Fitted Curves

The observed responses, the responses fitted under hypothesis H (joined by a dashed line), and the responses fitted under hypothesis A (joined by a solid line) are plotted versus the degree-days scale:

```
> plot(DegreeDays,DryWeight,xlab="DegreeDays",ylab="dry weight",
      main="Growth of winter wheat tillers example",
      sub="Observed response")
> X<-seq(400,685,length=100)
> Y<-tiller.nl7$theta[1] *
        exp((tiller.nl7$theta[2]*X)**tiller.nl7$theta[3])
> lines(X,Y)
> Z<-tiller.nl2$theta[1]*exp(tiller.nl2$theta[2]*X)
> par (lty=2)
> lines (X,Z)
> par (lty=1)
```

(See Figure 3.5, page 76.)

Likelihood Ratio Test of H: $\theta_3 = 1$ against A: $\theta_3 \neq 1$

To be sure that the second model fits the tiller data better, we test hypothesis H: $\theta_3 = 1$ against the alternative A: $\theta_3 \neq 1$ using a likelihood ratio test. We calculate and display the statistic S_L (see Equation (3.14), page 71) and the 0.95 quantile of a χ^2 with one degree of freedom with which it should be compared:

```
> cat( "Sl:",
      dim(tiller)[1] * (tiller.nl2$loglik - tiller.nl7$loglik),
      "X2(0.95,1):",  qchisq(0.95,1), "\n\n")
```

Confidence Interval for θ_3 Using the Asymptotic Distribution of $\widehat{\theta}_3$

We calculate the confidence interval $\widehat{I}_N$ (see Equation (2.2), page 32, and Section 3.4.5, page 73) using the function **confidence**. We display the values of $\widehat{\theta}_3$, $\widehat{S}$, $\nu_{0.975}$, and $\widehat{I}_N$:

```
> tiller.In <- confidence(tiller.nl7)
>   # Print the results:
> cat("Estimated value of theta_3:", tiller.nl7$theta[3],"\n" )
> cat("Estimated value of S:", sqrt(tiller.nl7$as.var[3, 3]),"\n" )
> cat("nu_(0.975):", qnorm(0.975),"\n" )
> cat("Estimated value of In:",tiller.In$normal.conf.int[3,],"\n" )
```

Confidence Interval for θ_3 Using the Log-Likelihood Ratio

To calculate the confidence interval based on the log-likelihood ratio (see Section 3.4.5, page 73, and $\widehat{I}_S$ Section 3.5.1, page 76), we use the function conflike. We display the values of $\widehat{\theta}_3$, $\widehat{S}$, $\chi^1_{1,0.95}$, and $\widehat{I}_S$:

```
> cat("Estimated value of theta_3:", tiller.nl7$theta[3],"\n" )
> cat("Estimated value of S:", sqrt(tiller.nl7$as.var[3, 3]),"\n" )
> cat("X2(0.95,1):", qchisq(0.95, 1),"\n" )
> cat("Estimated value of Is:",
     conflike(tiller.nl7,parameter=3)$like.conf.int,"\n" )
```

(Results for this example are given in Section 3.5.1, page 74.)

The function conflike also allows us to carry out all of the steps of the calculation shown page 76.

Confidence Interval for θ_3 Using the Bootstrap Method

To calculate the confidence interval $\widehat{I}_B$ defined in Section (3.4.3), page 71, we use the function bootstrap. Several methods of bootstrap simulations are possible. Here, we choose wild.2, which means that pseudoerrors are obtained by multiplying the residuals by the independent random variables T defined at Equation (3.15), page 72.

To initialize the iterative process of bootstrap, nls2 must be called with the option renls2. We also set the option control so that intermediary results are not printed. Finally, we call the function delnls2 to destroy any internal structures:

```
> tiller.nl7 <- nls2(tiller, "tiller.exp.m7",
           list(theta.start = c(tiller.nl2$theta, 1), max.iters=500),
           control=list(freq=0), renls2=T)
> tiller.boot <- bootstrap( tiller.nl7, method="wild.2",
                        n.loops=500)
> delnls2()
```

We calculate the 2.5% and 97.5% quantiles of the $\widehat{T}^{\star,b}$, $b = 1, \ldots 500$, using the function quantile of S-Plus, and we display the values of $\widehat{\theta}_3$, $\widehat{S}$, $b_{0.025}$, $b_{0.975}$, and $\widehat{I}_B$:

```
> tiller.Tg <- (tiller.boot$pStar[,3]-tiller.nl7$theta[3])/
             sqrt(tiller.boot$var.pStar[,3])
> qu  <- quantile(tiller.Tg,probs=c(0.975,0.025))
> tiller.IntBoot <- tiller.nl7$theta[3]
       - qu*sqrt(tiller.nl7$as.var[3,3])
> cat("Estimated value of theta_3:", tiller.nl7$theta[3],"\n")
> cat("Estimated value of S:", sqrt(tiller.nl7$as.var[3,3]),"\n")
> cat("b_(0.025):", qu[2],"\n" )
> cat("b_(0.975):", qu[1],"\n" )
> cat("Estimated value of Ib:",
     tiller.nl7$theta[3] + qu[2]*sqrt(tiller.nl7$as.var[3,3],
     tiller.nl7$theta[3] + qu[1]*sqrt(tiller.nl7$as.var[3,3],"\n")
```

Solubility of Peptides Example

The solubility of peptides example is a new example, introduced in this chapter. First we create a *data frame* to store the experimental data. Then we estimate the parameters with several models, and, finally, we calculate confidence intervals to compare them.

Creating the Data

The experimental data (see Table 3.2, page 64) are stored in a *data frame* called pept.d:

```
> RetTime <-c(
  3.6,   3.6,   6.7, 11.2, 20.0, 21.5,
 24.5, 29.2, 38.4, 40.4, 49.8, 59.6,
 64.2, 68.1, 72.7, 40.8, 52.7, 57.7,
 59.1, 61.7, 65.7, 28.3, 33.0, 40.0,
 44.5, 47.0, 63.1, 31.6, 40.1, 52.4,
 57.5, 23.8, 29.1, 30.0, 31.7, 23.1,
 42.7, 46.8, 16.8, 24.0, 31.1, 32.3,
 34.0, 34.7, 36.3, 39.3, 42.0, 44.4,
 45.0, 46.2, 49.0, 52.1, 55.4, 56.7,
 53.0, 0.0, 3.1,   4.2,   7.1, 9.0, 10.6,
 13.0, 14.2, 15.5, 38.3, 43.5, 45.9,
 47.5, 48.9, 55.6, 57.0, 59.2, 60.9, 34.3, 51.5)
> solubility  <-c(
 100, 100, 99, 105, 100, 84, 100, 99, 88, 48, 35, 0,
   0, 0, 0, 50, 2, 0, 0, 0, 0, 104, 89, 56, 10, 0, 0,
  91, 32, 2, 4, 100, 85, 95, 100, 95, 85, 95, 101, 100,
 107, 84, 92, 94, 97, 95, 0, 51, 0, 70, 63, 1, 0, 0,
   0, 82, 102, 100, 100, 95, 106, 93, 107, 98, 92, 48,
  90, 65, 34, 8, 0, 1, 0, 100, 0)
> pept.d <- data.frame(RetTime , solubility)
```

Plot of the Observed Percentage of Solubility Versus the Retention Time

We plot the observed responses versus the retention time using the graphical function pldnls2:

```
> pldnls2(pept.d, response.name="solubility", X.name="RetTime",
         title="Solubility of peptides example",
         sub="observed response")
```

(See Figure 3.3, page 65.)

Find Initial Values for the Regression Parameters

To find reasonable starting values for the parameters, we make a first estimation using ordinary least squares estimators and assume constant variance. This model is described in a file called pept.m1:

```
% model pept.m1
resp solubility;
varind RetTime;
aux a1;
parresp  ed50, sl ;
subroutine ;
begin
a1 = 1 + exp (sl*(RetTime-ed50)) ;
solubility = 100. /a1 ;
end
```

We apply function **nls2** to estimate the parameters:

```
> pept.nl1<-nls2(pept.d, "pept.m1",
     list(theta.start=c(1,1), max.iters=100))
```

Estimation under Hypothesis A

To see whether a constant term in the variance is necessary to describe correctly the variability of the data, we first try a variance model with a constant term. We describe it in a file called **pept.m3**:

```
% model pept.m3
resp solubility;
varind RetTime;
var v;
aux a1;
parresp  ed50, sl ;
parvar h;
subroutine ;
begin
a1 = 1 + exp (sl*(RetTime-ed50)) ;
solubility = 100. /a1 ;
v= 1 + h*solubility*(100.-solubility)  ;
end
```

We call **nls2** and display the results:

```
>  pept.c3 <- list(theta.start=pept.nl1$theta,
                  beta.start=0)
>  pept.nl3<-nls2(pept.d, "pept.m3", stat.ctx= pept.c3)
>     # Print the results
> cat("Summary of pept.nl3:\n")
> summary( pept.nl3)
```

We plot the observed and fitted responses versus the retention time using the graphical function **plfit**. The option **wanted** specifies the requested plot; the observed and fitted values are plotted against the independent variable:

```
> plfit(pept.nl3, wanted=list(X.OF=T),
        title="Solubility of peptides example",
        sub="Observed and fitted response")
```

(See Figure 3.8, page 80.)

Estimation under Hypothesis H

Now we try a variance model without a constant term. This model is described in a file called pept.m2:

```
% model pept.m2
resp solubility;
varind RetTime;
var v;
aux a1;
parresp ed50, sl ;
subroutine ;
begin
a1 = 1 + exp (sl*(RetTime-ed50)) ;
solubility = 100. /a1 ;
v= solubility*(100.-solubility) ;
end
```

The parameters of this model are estimated using the function nls2:

```
> pept.nl2<-nls2(pept.d, "pept.m2",pept.nl1$theta)
```

Likelihood Ratio Test of the Existence of a Constant Term in the Variance Model

We calculate and display the test statistic S_L (see Equation (3.14), page 71) and the 0.95 quantile of a χ^2 with one degree of freedom, with which S_L should be compared:

```
> cat( "S1:",
    75 * (pept.nl2$loglik - pept.nl3$loglik),
    "X2(0.95,1):",  qchisq(0.95,1), "\n\n")
```

Plots of the Fitted Curves

The observed responses, the responses fitted under hypothesis H (joined by a dashed line), and the responses fitted under hypothesis A (joined by a solid line) are plotted versus the retention time:

```
> plot(RetTime,solubility,xlab="retention time",ylab="solubility",
        main="Solubility of peptides example",
        sub="Observed and fitted response")
> X<-seq(-1,75,length=100)
> Y<-100/(1+exp(pept.nl3$theta[2]*(X-pept.nl3$theta[1])))
> lines(X,Y)
> Z<-100/(1+exp(pept.nl2$theta[2]*(X-pept.nl2$theta[1])))
> par (lty=2)
> lines (X,Z)
> par (lty=1)
```

(See Figure 3.9, page 81.)

Confidence Interval for θ_2 Using the Log-Likelihood Ratio

We calculate a confidence interval based on the log-likelihood ratio (see Section 3.4.5, page 73, and $\widehat{I}_S$ Section 3.5.1, page 76) using the function `conflike`. We display the values of $\widehat{\theta}_2$, $\widehat{S}$, $\chi^1_{1,0.95}$, and $\widehat{I}_S$:

```
> pept.conflike _ conflike(pept.nl3, parameter = 2)
>   # Print the results
> cat("Estimated value of theta_2:", pept.nl3$theta[2],"\n" )
> cat("Estimated value of S:", sqrt(pept.nl3$as.var[2, 2]),"\n" )
> cat("X2(0.95,1):", qchisq(0.95, 1),"\n" )
> cat("Estimated value of Is:", pept.conflike$like.conf.int,"\n" )
```

Confidence Interval for θ_2 Using the Wald Statistic, Based on the Maximum Likelihood Estimator

To calculate a confidence interval for θ_2 using the Wald statistic (see Section 3.4.4, page 72), we apply the function `confidence`. We display the values of $\widehat{\theta}_2$, $\widehat{S}$, $\nu_{0.975}$, and $\widehat{I}_{\mathcal{N}}$:

```
> pept.conf_confidence(pept.nl3)
>    # Print the results:
> cat("Estimated value of theta_2:",pept.conf$psi[2],"\n" )
> cat("Estimated value of S:", pept.conf$std.error[2],"\n" )
> cat("nu_(0.975):", qnorm(0.975),"\n" )
> cat("Estimated value of In:",pept.conf$normal.conf.int[2,], "\n" )
```

Confidence Interval for θ_2 Using the Wald Statistic, Based on the Three-Step Alternate Method

The alternate method is included in the function `nls2`: Option `method` introduces the three requested methods. They are as follows; `OLST`, ordinary least square, to estimate the parameters θ; `MLSB`, modified least square, to estimate the parameters β; and `MLST`, modified least square, to reestimate the parameters θ.

We display the values of the parameters and the asymptotic covariance matrix estimated at the last step:

```
> pept.nl8<-nls2(pept.d, "pept.m3", pept.c3,
    method=c("OLST","MLSB","MLST"))
>   # Print the results
> cat("Estimated value of the parameters theta:\n")
> print(pept.nl8$step3$theta)
> cat("Estimated value of the parameters beta:\n",
    pept.nl8$step3$beta[1], pept.nl8$step3$sigma2)
> cat("\nEstimated value of the asymptotic covariance matrix:\n")
> print(pept.nl8$step3$as.var[1:2, 1:2])
```

Plots of the Results

The observed responses, the responses fitted by the three-step alternate method (joined by a dashed line), and the responses fitted by the maximum likelihood method (joined by a solid line) are plotted versus the retention time:

```
> plot(RetTime,solubility,
        xlab="retention time",ylab="solubility",
        main="Solubility of peptides example",
        sub="Observed and fitted response")
> X<-seq(-1,75,length=100)
> Y<-100/(1+exp(pept.nl3$theta[2]*(X-pept.nl3$theta[1])))
> Z<-100/(1+exp(pept.nl8$step3$theta[2]*(X-pept.nl2$theta[1])))
> lines(X,Y)
> par (lty=2)
> lines (X,Z)
> par (lty=1)
```

(See Figure 3.10, page 82.)

Confidence Interval for θ_2 Based on Results of the Three-Step Method

Using the function `confidence`, we compute the confidence interval based on the Wald statistic from the results of estimation by the alternate method. We display the values of $\widehat{\theta}_2$, $\widehat{S}$, $\nu_{0.975}$, and $\widehat{I}'_{\mathcal{N}}$:

```
> pept.In <- confidence(pept.nl8)
>       # Print the results
> cat("Estimated value of theta_2:",coef(pept.nl8)$theta[2],"\n" )
> cat("Estimated value of S:", coef(pept.nl8)$std.error[2],"\n" )
> cat("nu_(0.975):", qnorm(0.975),"\n" )
> cat("Estimated value of In:",pept.In$normal.conf.int[2,],"\n" )
```

We display the log-likelihood values calculated by both methods to compare them:

```
> cat("Loglikelihood values:",
     -(pept.nl3$loglik*75/2), -(pept.nl8$step3$loglik*75/2),"\n" )
```

(Results for this example are given in Section 3.5.2, page 78.)

4

Diagnostics of Model Misspecification

In Section 1.2, we denoted the true regression relationship between Y and x by $\mu(x)$, and we noted that $\mu(x)$ is generally unknown, although in practice it is approximated by a parametric function $f(x, \theta)$. Because we use this f to make some statistical inferences, however, we must be able to determine whether our choice of f is accurate.

We can detect model misspecification by examining the data with the results of the estimation. It is an iterative procedure. The goal is to check if the assumptions on which the analysis is based are fairly accurate and to detect and correct any existing *model misspecification*. For this purpose we present two types of tools in this chapter: Graphics and tests. We apply each of these to some of our previously cited examples.

4.1 Problem Formulation

Let us recall the assumptions: We observe (Y_{ij}, x_i), $i = 1, \ldots k$, $j = 1, n_i$. We consider the parametric functions f and g such that

$$Y_{ij} = f(x_i, \theta) + \varepsilon_{ij},$$
$$\mathrm{Var}\,\varepsilon_{ij} = g(x_i, \sigma^2, \theta, \tau).$$

We assume that the errors ε_{ij} are independent for all (i, j).

Then we estimate the parameters. Before we describe how to detect misspecifications, let us give the list of assumptions that these procedures need to check:

- The regression function f is correct. The true regression function $\mu(x)$ should satisfy $\mu(x) = f(x, \theta)$ for one value of θ in Θ and for all values of x. If this condition exists, it implies that the errors are centered variables: $\mathrm{E}\varepsilon_{ij} = 0$. If not, $\mathrm{E}Y_{ij} = \mu(x_i)$ and $\mathrm{E}\varepsilon_{ij} = \mu(x_i) - f(x_i, \theta)$, which is different from zero for at least some values of x_i, $i = 1, \ldots n$. In this latter case, the *classical asymptotic results* stated in Section 2.3 are no longer valid.

- The variance function is correct. The most frequent mistake made in modeling the variance function is to assume that the variance of errors is constant, $\operatorname{Var}\varepsilon_{ij} = \sigma^2$, when, in actuality, heteroscedasticity exists, $\operatorname{Var}\varepsilon_{ij} = \sigma_i^2$. In that case, when the number of observations tends to infinity, the variance of $V_{\widehat{\theta}}^{-1/2}(\widehat{\theta} - \theta)$ is different from the identity matrix.
- The observations are *independent*. Suppose that we are interested in the growth of some characteristic as a function of time. We observe the response Y_i at time t_i for one individual, for $i = 1, \ldots n$. Generally, the relationship between the growth and the time, say $f(t, \theta)$, is a smooth function of t. If, however, the t_i are such that the $t_{i+1} - t_i$ are small with respect to the variations of the growth, correlations exist between the variables Y_i. The observations thus are not independent, and the results of Section 2.3 cannot be applied, as we will see in Section 4.2.5.

4.2 Diagnostics of Model Misspecifications with Graphics

Graphic of Fitted and Observed Values

If the Y_i satisfy $\mathrm{E}Y_i = f(x_i, \theta)$, then the *fitted values* $f(x_i, \widehat{\theta})$ estimate the expectation of the Y_i. To detect a bad choice of the regression function, we use either a plot of fitted $f(x_i, \widehat{\theta})$ and observed Y_i values versus x_i or a plot of fitted versus observed values. These graphics tools offer a simple way to look simultaneously at data and fitted values.

Graphics of Residuals and Standardized Residuals

If the choice of the regression function is correct, then the

$$\varepsilon_{ij} = Y_{ij} - f(x_i, \theta), \text{ for } i = 1, \ldots k, \quad j = 1, \ldots n_i$$

are centered independent variables; and if $\operatorname{Var} \varepsilon_{ij} = \sigma_i^2$, the standardized errors

$$e_{ij} = \frac{Y_{ij} - f(x_i, \theta)}{\sigma_i}, \text{ for } i = 1, \ldots k, \quad j = 1, \ldots n_i,$$

are centered independent variables with variance equal to 1. In the same way, if the variance function is $\sigma_i^2 = g(x_i, \sigma^2, \theta, \tau)$, then the

$$e_{ij} = \frac{Y_{ij} - f(x_i, \theta)}{\sqrt{g(x_i, \sigma^2, \theta, \tau)}}, \text{ for } i = 1, \ldots k, \quad j = 1, \ldots n_i,$$

are centered independent variables with variance equal to 1. A natural idea is to estimate the errors and standardized errors and then study their behavior. The *residuals*

$$\widehat{\varepsilon}_{ij} = Y_{ij} - f(x_i, \widehat{\theta})$$

and the *standardized residuals*

$$\widehat{e}_{ij} = \frac{Y_{ij} - f(x_i, \widehat{\theta})}{\widehat{\sigma}_i}$$

are estimates of the errors and standardized errors. Model misspecification usually is detected by examining the graphics of residuals. To detect a bad choice of the regression or variance functions, we use the graphics of $\widehat{\varepsilon}_{ij}$, $\widehat{e}_{ij}$, $|\widehat{\varepsilon}_{ij}|$, $|\widehat{e}_{ij}|$, $\widehat{\varepsilon}_{ij}^2$, $\widehat{e}_{ij}^2$ versus x_i, $f(x_i, \widehat{\theta})$, or $g(x_i, \widehat{\sigma}^2, \widehat{\theta}, \widehat{\tau})$. If $n_i = 1$, the graphic of $\widehat{\varepsilon}_i$ versus $\widehat{\varepsilon}_{i-1}$ is convenient to detect some correlation between errors.

4.2.1 Pasture Regrowth Example: Estimation Using a Concave-Shaped Curve and Plot for Diagnostics

Let us again consider the pasture regrowth example using a concave-shaped curve for the function f in place of function (1.2).

Model The regression function is

$$f(x, \theta) = \frac{\theta_2 + \theta_1 x}{\theta_3 + x}, \tag{4.1}$$

and the variances are homogeneous: $\text{Var}(\varepsilon_i) = \sigma^2$.

Method The parameters are estimated by minimizing the sum of squares, $C(\theta)$; see Equation (1.10).

Results

Parameters	Estimated Values
θ_1	358.0
θ_2	−1326.0
θ_3	301.5
σ^2	6.802

Figure 4.1 shows that this regression function badly estimates the decreasing speed; moreover, the estimated value of θ_1, $\widehat{\theta}_1 = 358$ is not in accordance with the expected value (the graphic of observed values suggests the presence of an upper asymptote at a value of yield close to 70). Thus, we reject this regression function.

4.2.2 Isomerization Example: Graphics for Diagnostic

Consider the graph of fitted versus observed values drawn in Figure 1.9. To make this graph easier to read, one can plot the first diagonal and then superimpose a curve joining the points after smoothing (see Figure 4.2).

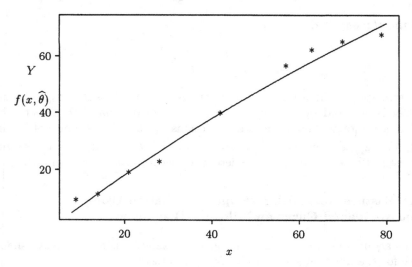

Figure 4.1. Pasture regrowth example: Graph of observed and adjusted values of the response after estimation using a concave-shaped curve

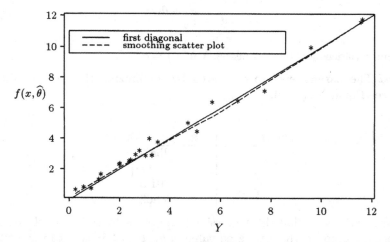

Figure 4.2. Isomerization example: Graph of adjusted versus observed values

Model The regression function is

$$f(x, \theta) = \frac{\theta_1 \theta_3 (P - I/1.632)}{1 + \theta_2 H + \theta_3 P + \theta_4 I},$$

where x is a three-dimensional variate, $x = (H, P, I)$, and the variances are homogeneous: $\mathrm{Var}(\varepsilon_i) = \sigma^2$.

Method The parameters are estimated by minimizing the sum of squares, $C(\theta)$; see Equation (1.10).

The plot shown in Figure 4.2 does not suggest any model misspecification: The points are well distributed around the first diagonal, and the smoothed scatter plot is close to the first diagonal.

Several plots of residuals are shown in Figure 4.3. None of these presents a particular structure; thus, we have no reason to suspect a departure from the hypotheses.

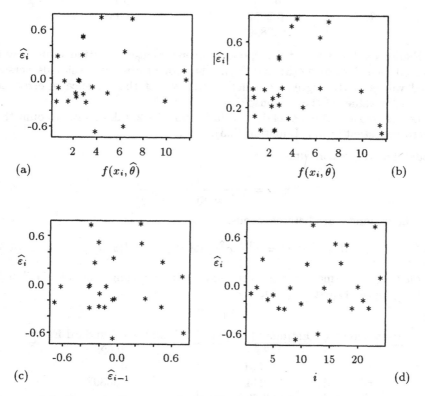

Figure 4.3. Isomerization example: Residual plots: (a) residuals versus the fitted reaction rate; (b) absolute residuals versus the fitted reaction rate; (c) residuals versus the preceding residual; and (d) residuals versus the residual order

4.2.3 Peptides Example: Graphics for Diagnostic

Let us consider the example described in Section 3.1.2, assuming a logistic curve for the regression function (see Equation (3.2)) and a constant variance.

Model The regression function is

$$f(x, \theta) = \frac{100}{1 + \exp\left(\theta_2\left(x - \theta_1\right)\right)},$$

and the variances are homogeneous: $\text{Var}(\varepsilon_i) = \sigma^2$.

Method The parameters are estimated by minimizing the sum of squares, $C(\theta)$; see Equation (1.10).

Results

Parameters	Estimated Values	Estimated Standard Error
θ_1	43.92	0.792
θ_2	0.2052	0.0316
σ^2	328.4	

Figure 4.4 shows that the response is overestimated for fitted values lower than 50 (see Figures 4.4(a) and (b)). The plot of absolute residuals versus fitted values of the regression function shows that the variance of errors is smaller for values of the response close to 0 or 100.

Let us consider the model defined in Section 3.1.2, taking into account the heteroscedasticity using Equation (3.3).

Model The regression function is

$$f(x, \theta) = \frac{100}{1 + \exp(\theta_2(x - \theta_1))}, \tag{4.2}$$

and the variances are heterogeneous:

$$g(x, \sigma^2, \theta, \tau) = \sigma^2 + \sigma^2 \tau f(x, \theta) \left[100 - f(x, \theta)\right]. \tag{4.3}$$

Method The parameters are estimated by maximizing the log-likelihood, $V(\theta, \sigma^2, \tau)$; see Equation (3.8).

Results

Parameters	Estimated Values	Estimated Standard Error
θ_1	43.93	0.628
θ_2	0.4331	0.0557
τ_1	0.02445	0.00897
σ^2	26.79	

Figure 4.5 shows that the results of the estimation differ from the preceding case when we assume homogeneous variances. The estimated values of the response are in better accordance with the observed values; see Figures 4.5(a) and (b). The estimated value of θ_2 is now equal to 0.4331, in place of 0.2052. Thus, the estimation of the maximum of the slope has increased, and the problem of overestimation for values of the response lower than 50 has disappeared. The interpretation of Figure 4.5(c) showing the absolute values of the standardized residuals versus the fitted responses is not as clear, however; if the variance function were well modeled, the points of this graph would not present any particular structure. We can only say that the structure of the points is not as pronounced as when we assumed a constant variance. We will return to this example in Section 4.4.

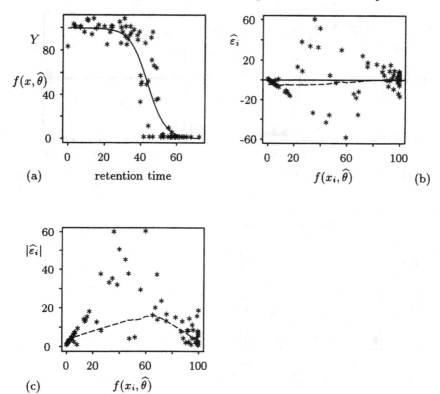

Figure 4.4. Peptides example: Plots of fitted values and residuals: (a) observed (∗) and fitted (line) values of solubility versus retention time; (b) residuals versus fitted values, the solid line is horizontal, passing through 0, and the dotted line is a curve joining the points after smoothing; and (c) absolute residuals versus fitted values, the dotted line is a curve joining the points after smoothing

4.2.4 Cortisol Assay Example: How to Choose the Variance Function Using Replications

Figure 1.3 suggests that we can model the relationship between the response and the log-dose using a symmetric sigmoidally shaped curve:

$$f(x, \theta) = \theta_1 + \frac{\theta_2 - \theta_1}{1 + \exp(\theta_3 + \theta_4 x)}.$$

This equation is similar to Equation (1.3) with $\theta_5 = 1$. To illustrate a frequent mistake, let us see what happens if we hypothesize that the variance is constant rather than heteroscedastic.

Model The regression function is

$$f(x, \theta) = \theta_1 + \frac{\theta_2 - \theta_1}{1 + \exp(\theta_3 + \theta_4 x)},$$

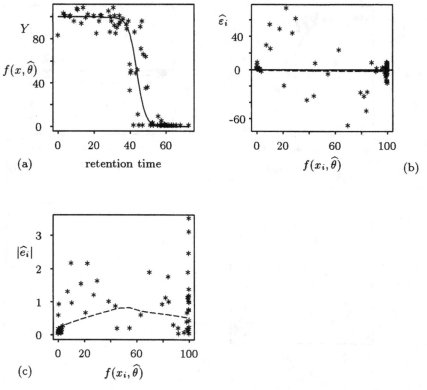

Figure 4.5. Peptides example: Plots of fitted values and residuals taking into account heteroscedasticity: (a) observed and fitted values of solubility versus retention time; (b) residuals versus fitted values, the solid line is horizontal, passing through 0 and the dotted line is a curve joining the points after smoothing; and (c) absolute standardized residuals versus fitted values, the dotted line is a curve joining the points after smoothing

and the variances are homogeneous: $\text{Var}(\varepsilon_i) = \sigma^2$.

Method The parameters are estimated by minimizing the sum of squares, $C(\theta)$; see Equation (1.10).

Results

Parameters	Estimated Values	Estimated Standard Error
θ_1	175.46	19.1
θ_2	2777.3	18.1
θ_3	2.0125	0.065
θ_4	2.6872	0.068
σ^2	3085	

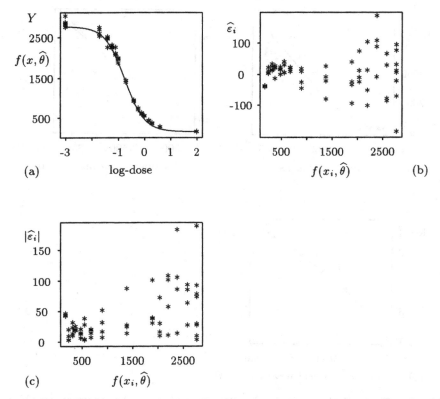

Figure 4.6. Cortisol assay example: Plots of fitted values and residuals under the hypothesis of a symmetric sigmoidally shaped regression function and of a constant variance: (a) observed and fitted values of counts versus the log-dose; (b) residuals versus fitted values; and (c) absolute residuals versus fitted values

The graph of absolute residuals versus fitted values of the response (Figure 4.6) clearly shows that the dispersion of the residuals varies with the values of the fitted response. This suggests that Var $\varepsilon_{ij} = \sigma_i^2$.

In this example, the experimental design allows us to calculate the s_i^2 (see Equation (1.4)), which estimates VarY_{ij} independent of the estimated regression function. Graphs of s_i^2, or functions of s_i^2 versus $Y_{i\bullet}$, can be used to choose the variance function g or to confirm the presence of heteroscedasticity, as we see in Figure 4.7.

The graphs presented in Figure 4.7 show that the relation between s_i and $Y_{i\bullet}$ is nearly linear (see Figure 4.7(b)), thereby suggesting that the variance of the response could be assumed proportional to the squared response. It follows that the function $g(x_i, \sigma^2, \theta) = \sigma^2 f^2(x_i, \theta)$ is a good candidate for the variance function. Another choice could be $g(x_i, \sigma^2, \theta, \tau) = \sigma^2 f^\tau(x_i, \theta)$, where τ is a parameter to be estimated; see Chapter 3.

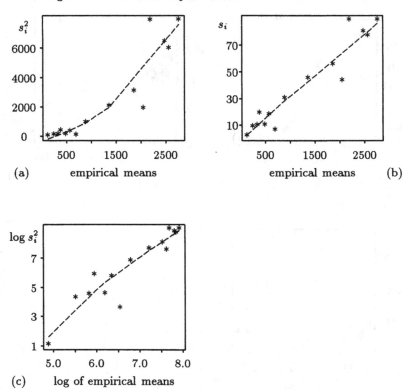

Figure 4.7. Cortisol assay example: Plots of empirical variances versus empirical means; a curve joining the points after smoothing (broken line) is superimposed on each plot: (a) empirical variances versus empirical means; (b) square root of the empirical variances versus the empirical means; and (c) logarithm of the empirical variances versus the logarithm of empirical means

Now, let us again estimate the parameters, this time under the assumption $\operatorname{Var}Y_{ij} = \sigma^2 f^2(x_i, \theta)$.

Model The regression function is

$$f(x_i, \theta) = \theta_1 + \frac{\theta_2 - \theta_1}{1 + \exp(\theta_3 + \theta_4 x_i)}, \tag{4.4}$$

and the variances are heterogeneous:

$$\operatorname{Var}(\varepsilon_{ij}) = \sigma^2 f^2(x_i, \theta).$$

Method The parameters are estimated by maximizing the log-likelihood, $V(\theta, \sigma^2, \tau)$; see Equation (3.8).

Results

Parameters	Estimated Values	Estimated Standard Error
θ_1	137.15	2.64
θ_2	2855.8	33.9
θ_3	1.8543	0.021
θ_4	2.3840	0.034
σ^2	0.001614	

From the plots presented in Figure 4.8, we can see that the points on the graph of absolute standardized residuals versus fitted values of the response (Figure 4.8(c)) are nearly uniformly distributed. This confirms the choice of the variance function. On the other hand, the plot of standardized residuals shows that the response is overestimated for low values (between 500 and 1500) and underestimated between 1500 and 2500. This result suggests that the maximum of decrease is closer to the upper asymptote, and it points us to the generalized logistic model in Equation (1.3).

Model The regression function is

$$f(x_i, \theta) = \theta_1 + \frac{\theta_2 - \theta_1}{(1 + \exp(\theta_3 + \theta_4 x_i))^{\theta_5}}, \tag{4.5}$$

and the variances are heterogeneous:

$$\mathrm{Var}(\varepsilon_{ij}) = \sigma^2 f^2(x_i, \theta).$$

Method The parameters are estimated by maximizing the log-likelihood, $V(\theta, \sigma^2, \tau)$; see Equation (3.8).

Results

Parameters	Estimated Values	Estimated Standard Error
θ_1	133.42	1.94
θ_2	2758.7	26.3
θ_3	3.2011	0.223
θ_4	3.2619	0.159
θ_5	0.6084	0.041
σ^2	0.0008689	

The graphics presented in Figure 4.9 do not suggest any model misspecification.

4.2.5 Trajectory of Roots of Maize: How to Detect Correlations in Errors

When *correlations* exist between the observations, the graphic of the residuals $\widehat{\varepsilon}_i$ versus $\widehat{\varepsilon}_{i-1}$ is a good tool to detect this lack of independence. Let us introduce a new example to illustrate this case.

The trajectory of roots is projected onto a vertical plane; the scientist then draws this projection to create a data set by numerization [TP90]. The

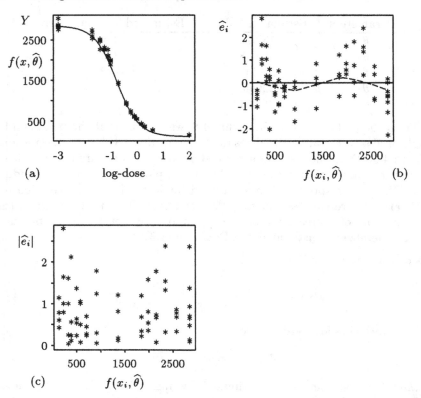

Figure 4.8. Cortisol assay example: Plots of fitted values and standardized residuals under the hypothesis of a symmetric sigmoidally shaped regression function and heteroscedasticity: (a) observed and fitted values of counts versus the log-dose; (b) standardized residuals versus fitted values, a curve joining the points after smoothing (broken line) is superimposed; and (c) absolute standardized residuals versus fitted values

variable Y is the distance between the root and the vertical axis running through the foot of the plant, and x is the depth in the ground. The scientist can pick up as many points as necessary to describe the trajectory of each root, as shown in Figure 4.10.

A nonlinear regression model describes this phenomenon by modeling the relation between Y and x with the function $f(x, \theta) = \theta_1(1 - \exp(-\theta_2 x))$.

Model The regression function is

$$f(x, \theta) = \theta_1(1 - exp(-\theta_2 x)),$$

and the variances are homogeneous: $\mathrm{Var}(\varepsilon_i) = \sigma^2$.

Method The parameters are estimated by minimizing the sum of squares, $C(\theta)$; see Equation (1.10).

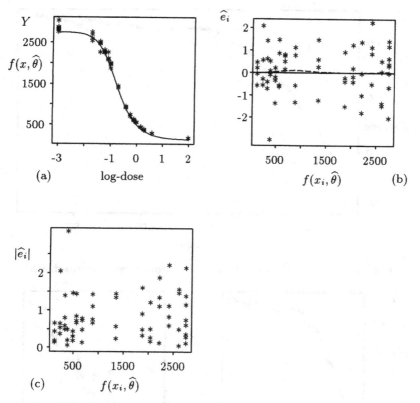

Figure 4.9. Cortisol assay example: Plots of fitted values and standardized residuals under the hypothesis of an asymmetric sigmoidally shaped regression function and heteroscedasticity: (a) observed and fitted values of counts versus the log-dose; (b) standardized residuals versus fitted values, a curve joining the points after smoothing (broken line) is superimposed; and (c) absolute standardized residuals versus fitted values

Results

Parameters	Estimated Values
θ_1	67.876
θ_2	0.05848

Figure 4.10 clearly shows that the quantities $Y_i - f(x_i, \theta)$ and $Y_j - f(x_j, \theta)$ are not independent when i and j are close to each other. Moreover, the points of the graph (see Figure 4.11(b)) of $\widehat{\varepsilon}_i$ versus $\widehat{\varepsilon}_{i-1}$ are distributed along the first diagonal. This distribution suggests that the correlation between the observations could be modeled by an autoregressive model: $\varepsilon_i = \rho\varepsilon_{i-1} + \eta_i$, where $\rho \in [-1, 1]$ is a parameter, generally unknown, and η_i for $i = 1, \ldots n$ are independent random variables with expectation 0 and variance σ^2. Models taking into account correlated observations are not treated in

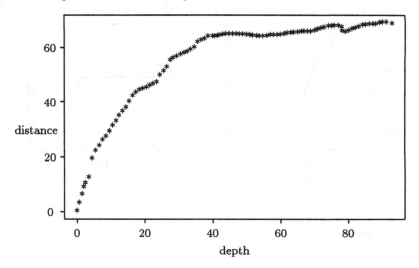

Figure 4.10. Trajectory of roots of maize: Distance versus depth

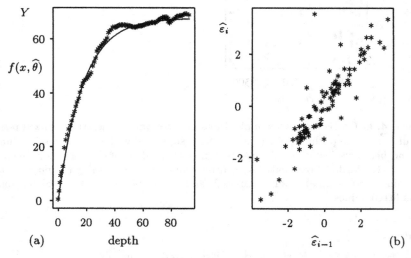

Figure 4.11. Trajectory of roots of maize: (a) observed and adjusted values of the response; and (b) residual versus preceding residual

this book, but interested users will find several publications on that subject, including Glasbey [Gla80] and White and Domowitz [WD84].

4.2.6 What Can We Say About the Experimental Design?

Obvious links exist between the choice of the regression function and the choice of the *experimental design*, $x_1, x_2, \ldots x_k$. For example, k must be greater than p.

Consider again the cortisol example. Intuitively, we know that if we suppress the observations corresponding to a logarithm of the dose between -1 and 0, the parameters θ_3, θ_4, and θ_5 will not be estimated *easily*. The estimating procedure will not converge, the estimated standard error of the estimated parameters will be very large with respect to their values, or the estimated values of the parameters will be aberrant for the scientist.

In this case, one must verify if the values of x and the regression function are in accord. For this purpose we use *sensitivity functions* to describe the link between f and x.

Let $f(x, \theta)$ be the regression function, where θ is the vector with p components θ_a, $a = 1, \ldots p$. The sensitivity function for parameter θ_a is the derivative of f with respect to θ_a:

$$\Phi_a(x, \theta) = \frac{\partial f}{\partial \theta_a}(x, \theta).$$

Consider that the value of x is fixed; thus, if the absolute value of $\Phi_a(x, \theta)$ is small, the variations of $f(x, \theta)$ are small when θ_a varies. It follows that in order to estimate θ_a accurately, we must choose x such that the absolute value of $\Phi_a(x, \theta)$ is large.

Let us illustrate this procedure with a simulated data set.

Data The data are simulated in the following way. Let $\mu(x) = 1 - \exp(-x)$, and let ε be a centered normal variable with variance 25×10^{-4}. The values of x are chosen in the following way: $x_i = i/10$ for $i = 1, \ldots 10$. The observations Y_i are defined as $Y_i = \mu(x_i) + \varepsilon_i$, where the ε_i, $i = 1, \ldots 10$, are independent variables with the same distribution as ε.

x	0.1	0.2	0.3	0.4	0.5
Y	0.1913	0.0737	0.2702	0.4270	0.2968
x	0.6	0.7	0.8	0.9	1.0
Y	0.4474	0.4941	0.5682	0.5630	0.6636

Model The regression function is

$$f(x, \theta) = \theta_1(1 - \exp(-\theta_2 x)),$$

and the variances are homogeneous: $\mathrm{Var}(\varepsilon_i) = \sigma^2$.

Method The parameters are estimated by minimizing the sum of squares, $C(\theta)$; see Equation (1.10).

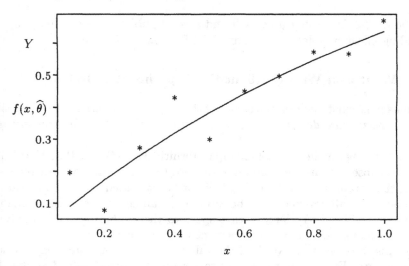

Figure 4.12. Simulated example: First data set, graph of simulated data and fitted values of the response

Results

Parameters	Estimated Values	Estimated Standard Errors
θ_1	1.1007	0.49
θ_2	0.8654	0.54
σ^2	0.00418	

The estimated standard errors are very large. Using Equation (2.3), we find that the confidence interval for θ_1, with asymptotic level 95%, is $[0.13; 2.07]$, and for θ_2 it is $[-0.19; 1.93]$. The interval for θ_2 contains 0, which is an unacceptable value in this example.

Looking at Figure 4.12, we can posit that the estimates would be more accurate with a wider interval of variations for x. To quantify this remark, let us look at the plot of sensitivity functions.

The functions Φ_a are defined as follows:

$$\Phi_1(x, \theta) = 1 - \exp(-\theta_2 x),$$
$$\Phi_2(x, \theta) = \theta_1 x \exp(-\theta_2 x).$$

Generally, the value of θ is unknown and the functions Φ_a are calculated in $\widehat{\theta}$.

Figure 4.13 shows the plot of sensitivity functions $\Phi_1(x, \widehat{\theta})$ and $\Phi_2(x, \widehat{\theta})$. We see that median values of x, say between 0.5 and 2, contribute to the estimation of θ_2 with high accuracy, while greater values of x contribute to the estimation of θ_1.

Now, let us see what happens with more appropriate values of x.

Data The data are now simulated in the following way. The values of x are chosen in the interval $[0.1; 4.6]$. The observations Y_i are defined as $Y_i = \mu(x_i) + \varepsilon_i$,

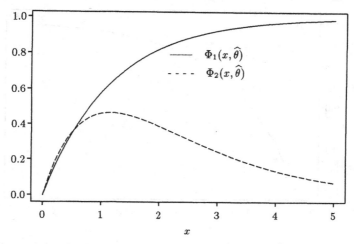

Figure 4.13. Simulated example: Graph of sensitivity functions calculated in $\widehat{\theta}$ versus x

where the ε_i, $i = 1, \ldots 10$, are independent variables with the same distribution as ε.

x	0.1	0.6	1.1	1.6	2.1
Y	0.1913	0.3436	0.6782	0.8954	0.7809
x	2.6	3.1	3.6	4.1	4.6
Y	0.9220	0.9457	0.9902	0.9530	1.0215

Model The regression function is

$$f(x, \theta) = \theta_1(1 - \exp(-\theta_2 x)),$$

and the variances are homogeneous: $\mathrm{Var}(\varepsilon_i) = \sigma^2$.

Method The parameters are estimated by minimizing the sum of squares, $C(\theta)$; see Equation (1.10).

Results

Parameters	Estimated Values	Estimated Standard Errors
θ_1	1.1006	0.04
θ_2	0.9512	0.14

As expected, the estimated standard errors are smaller than they were in the first data set. Comparing Figures 4.14 and 4.12 clearly shows that the experimental design in the second data set allows us to estimate the asymptote θ_1 better.

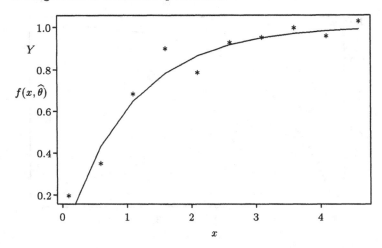

Figure 4.14. Simulated example: Second data set, graph of simulated data and fitted value of the response

4.3 Diagnostics of Model Misspecifications with Tests

4.3.1 RIA of Cortisol: Comparison of Nested Models

In some situations it is easy to find possible alternatives to the regression function or the variance function. For example, if we choose a symmetric sigmoidally shaped curve for the cortisol data, it is reasonable to wonder if an asymmetric curve would not be more appropriate.

Let us consider the models defined in Equations (4.4) and (4.5). If we suspect an asymmetry of the curve, we can test hypothesis H: $\theta_5 = 1$ against the alternative A: $\theta_5 \neq 1$. Let us apply a likelihood ratio test. Let $\widehat{\theta}_H$ be the estimator of θ under hypothesis H and $\widehat{\sigma}_H^2 f^2(x_i, \widehat{\theta}_H)$ be the estimator of $\mathrm{Var}(\varepsilon_{ij})$. In the same way, let us define $\widehat{\sigma}_A^2 f^2(x_i, \widehat{\theta}_A)$ as the estimator of $\mathrm{Var}(\varepsilon_{ij})$ under the alternative A. The test statistic

$$S_L = \sum_{i=1}^{k} \log \widehat{\sigma}_H^2 f^2(x_i, \widehat{\theta}_H) - \sum_{i=1}^{k} \log \widehat{\sigma}_A^2 f^2(x_i, \widehat{\theta}_A)$$

equals 39, which must be compared to the 0.95 quantile of a χ^2 with one degree of freedom. The hypothesis of a symmetric regression function is rejected.

The following section presents a likelihood ratio test based on the comparison between the considered model and a bigger model defined when the response is observed with replications.

4.3.2 Tests Using Replications

Let us return to the general nonlinear regression model with replications. We assume that for each value of x, x_i, $i = 1, \ldots k$, the number n_i of observed values of the response is large, greater than 4 for example. We choose a regression function, f, and carry out the estimation of the parameters. Let H be the considered model:

$$\left.\begin{array}{r} Y_{ij} = f(x_i, \theta) + \varepsilon_{ij} \\ \text{Var}(\varepsilon_{ij}) = \sigma^2, \ \text{E}(\varepsilon_{ij}) = 0 \end{array}\right\} .$$

$\widehat{\theta}_H$ is the estimation of θ and $\widehat{\sigma}_H^2$ is the estimation of σ^2. Under H, we estimate $p + 1$ parameters.

H can be considered as a model nested in a more general one, denoted by A_1, defined in the following way:

$$\left.\begin{array}{r} Y_{ij} = \mu_i + \varepsilon_{ij} \\ \text{Var}(\varepsilon_{ij}) = \sigma^2, \ \text{E}(\varepsilon_{ij}) = 0 \end{array}\right\} .$$

Now the parameters to be estimated are $\mu_1, \ldots \mu_k$ and σ^2, that is, $k + 1$ parameters. The presence of replications in each x_i allows us to estimate μ_i by the empirical mean $Y_{i\bullet}$ and to build a *goodness-of-fit test* of hypothesis H against the alternative A_1 as in Section 2.3.3 or 3.4.2. The test statistic

$$S_L = n \log C(\widehat{\theta}_H) - n \log \sum_{i=1}^{k} n_i s_i^2$$

is asymptotically distributed as a χ^2 with $k - p$ degrees of freedom.

If the test is not significant, we have no reason to reject the regression function f.

By modifying A_1, one may also test the hypothesis of homogeneous variances. Let A_2 be defined by:

$$\left.\begin{array}{r} Y_{ij} = \mu_i + \varepsilon_{ij} \\ \text{Var}(\varepsilon_{ij}) = \sigma_i^2, \ \text{E}(\varepsilon_{ij}) = 0 \end{array}\right\} .$$

Under the model A_2, we estimate $2k$ parameters. The μ_i are estimated by empirical means, and the σ_i^2 are estimated by empirical variances, denoted by s_i^2. The test statistic

$$S_L = n \log \widehat{\sigma}_H^2 - \sum_{i=1}^{k} n_i \log s_i^2,$$

where $\widehat{\sigma}_H^2 = C(\widehat{\theta}_H)/n$ is asymptotically distributed as a χ^2 with $2k - p - 1$ degrees of freedom.

This test is easily extended to the case of heterogeneous variances under the model H. Let the considered model H be the following:

$$\left.\begin{array}{r} Y_{ij} = f(x_i, \theta) + \varepsilon_{ij} \\ \text{Var}(\varepsilon_{ij}) = g(x_i, \sigma^2, \theta, \tau), \ \text{E}(\varepsilon_{ij}) = 0 \end{array}\right\} .$$

Under H, we estimate $p + q + 1$ parameters (p for θ, q for τ, and 1 for σ^2). The test statistic

$$\mathcal{S}_{\mathrm{L}} = \sum_{i=1}^{k} n_i \log \widehat{\sigma}_{\mathrm{H}}^2 g(x_i, \widehat{\theta}_{\mathrm{H}}) - \sum_{i=1}^{k} n_i \log s_i^2$$

is asymptotically distributed as a χ^2 with $2k - p - q - 1$ degrees of freedom.

We illustrate this method based on replications using the cortisol assay example and the ovocytes example.

4.3.3 Cortisol Assay Example: Misspecification Tests Using Replications

Let us consider again the model H, where the regression function is assumed symmetric and the variance is assumed proportional to the squared expectation.

Model The regression function is defined by Equation (4.4), and the variances are heterogeneous:
$$\mathrm{Var}(\varepsilon_{ij}) = \sigma^2 f^2(x_i, \theta).$$

Method The parameters are estimated by maximizing the log-likelihood, $V(\theta, \sigma^2, \tau)$; see Equation (3.8).

Results We test the model H against the alternative A_2. The test statistic $\mathcal{S}_{\mathrm{L}}$ equals 50. This number must be compared to 37, the 0.95 quantile of a χ^2 with 25 ($k = 15$, and the number of parameters to be estimated is 5, 4 for θ, and 1 for σ^2) degrees of freedom. Hypothesis H is rejected.

Let us see what happens if we take into account an asymmetry in the regression function.

Model The regression function is defined by Equation (4.5), and the variances are heterogeneous:
$$\mathrm{Var}(\varepsilon_{ij}) = \sigma^2 f^2(x_i, \theta).$$

Method The parameters are estimated by maximizing the log-likelihood, $V(\theta, \sigma^2, \tau)$; see Equation (3.8).

Results The test statistic $\mathcal{S}_{\mathrm{L}}$ equals 10.5, which must be compared to 36.4, the 0.95 quantile of a χ^2 with 24 degrees of freedom. Hypothesis H is not rejected. The analysis of graphics of residuals shown in Figure 4.8 is strengthened.

4.3.4 Ovocytes Example: Graphics of Residuals and Misspecification Tests Using Replications

Let us return to the ovocytes example treated in Section 1.4.4. Let H be the following model.

Model The regression function is

$$f(t, P_w, P_s) = \frac{1}{V_0}(V_w(t) + V_s(t) + V_x),$$

where V_w and V_s are solutions of Equation (1.8), and the variances are homogeneous: $\mathrm{Var}(\varepsilon_i) = \sigma^2$.

Method The parameters are estimated by minimizing the sum of squares, $C(\theta)$; see Equation (1.10).

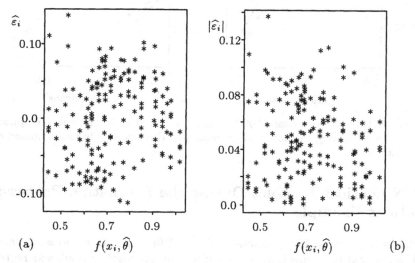

Figure 4.15. Ovocytes example: Plots of residuals: (a) residuals versus fitted volume; and (b) absolute standardized residuals versus fitted volume

Results Figure 4.15 shows the plots of residuals. The plots do not show any particular structure, except for a weak decrease of the absolute residuals when plotted against fitted values of the regression function. This behavior seems to be confirmed by the graph illustrating empirical variances versus empirical means (see Figure 4.16). However, this graph also shows that the empirical variances vary a lot.

Let us now look at the result of a misspecification test. The test statistic of hypothesis H against A_2, $\mathcal{S}_L$, equals 31, which must be compared to 71, the value of the 0.95 quantile of a χ^2 with 53 degrees of freedom (in that example, $k = 29$). Thus there is no reason to reject the hypothesis of a constant variance.

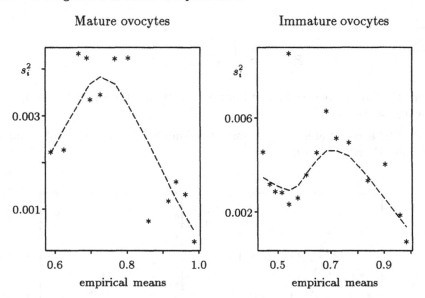

Figure 4.16. Ovocytes example: Graphs of empirical variances versus empirical means; a curve joining the points after smoothing (broken line) is superimposed on each plot

4.4 Numerical Troubles During the Estimation Process: Peptides Example

In this section we tackle a tedious problem: What should we do when faced with numerical problems during the estimation process? In nonlinear regression models, estimating the parameters needs an iterative *numerical process*. If the parameters are estimated by the least squares method, the numerical process minimizes the sum of squares $C(\theta)$ in Equation (1.10); if the parameters are estimated by maximizing the log-likelihood $V(\theta, \sigma^2, \tau)$ in Equation (3.8), the numerical process minimizes $-2V(\theta, \sigma^2, \tau)$. Starting from some initial values for the parameters to be estimated, the program calculates the criterion to minimize, and, using a specific algorithm (see, for example, [SW89]), it looks for new values of the parameter for which the value of the criterion to minimize is smaller. This procedure is stopped when a stopping criterion is small enough.

Generally, the user does not intervene in this iterative estimation process, because the methods used and their numerical options are automatically chosen by the program. Nevertheless, the user must choose the initial values of the parameters to start the iterative process.

All of the examples discussed in our book are treated using **nls2**; we did not have numerical difficulties for any of them during the iterative process for estimating the parameters. But as all users of nonlinear regression models know, numerical problems may appear, and, generally, the software's output is not informative enough to help and leaves the user puzzled.

Although it is difficult to list all of the reasons leading to a numerical problem, following are some troubleshooting procedures:

1. Check the data set and the model.
2. Try to run the program with another set of initial values.
3. Change the method used to estimate the parameters. This suggestion applies only in the case of heterogeneous variances when the parameters are estimated by minimizing $-2 \log V(\theta, \sigma^2, \tau)$. If the iterative process fails to converge, the user may run the program again, choosing another estimator, like a three-step alternate least squares (see Section (3.3.3)).
4. Change the parameterization of the regression function or the variance function. Sometimes, looking carefully at the behavior of the iterative estimation process, it appears that the problem comes from the estimation of one or two parameters. In some cases, the estimation process may run better by changing the parameterization of the model. For example, the following functions differ only in their parameterization:

$$f(x, \theta) = \exp\left(\theta_2(x - \theta_1)\right);$$
$$f(x, \alpha) = \exp(\alpha_1 + \alpha_2 x), \text{ with } \alpha_1 = -\theta_1\theta_2 \text{ and } \alpha_2 = \theta_2;$$
$$f(x, \beta) = \beta_1 \exp \beta_2 x, \text{ with } \beta_1 = \exp(-\theta_1\theta_2) \text{ and } \beta_2 = \theta_2;$$
$$f(x, \gamma) = \gamma_1 \gamma_2^x, \text{ with } \gamma_1 = \exp(-\theta_1\theta_2) \text{ and } \gamma_2 = \exp \theta_2.$$

5. Change the model. For example, we chose the Weibull model to represent a sigmoidally shaped curve in the pasture regrowth example, but several other models are available:

$$f_1(x, \theta) = \theta_1 \exp\left(\theta_2/(x + \theta_3)\right);$$
$$f_2(x, \theta) = \theta_1 \exp\left(-\exp(\theta_2 - \theta_3 x)\right);$$
$$f_3(x, \theta) = \theta_1 + \theta_2/\left(1 + \exp(\theta_3 - \theta_4 x)\right).$$

A list of nonlinear regression models can be found in the book by Ratkowsky [Rat89].

Let us illustrate some of these remarks with our peptides example by again examining the choice of variance function. To take into account the fact that the variability is greater when the peptide is fully soluble than when it is nonsoluble, we propose to generalize Equation (4.3) to the following:

$$\sigma_i^2 = \sigma^2 + \sigma^2 \tau_1 f(x_i, \theta) \left[100 + \tau_2 - f(x_i, \theta)\right] = g\left(x_i, \theta, \sigma^2, \tau_1, \tau_2\right).$$

When x equals 0, $g\left(x_i, \theta, \sigma^2, \tau_1, \tau_2\right)$ equals $\sigma^2(1 + 100\tau_1\tau_2)$ and when x tends to infinity, $g\left(x_i, \theta, \sigma^2, \tau_1, \tau_2\right)$ tends to σ^2. Let us estimate the parameters with this new model.

Model The regression function is

$$f(x, \theta) = \frac{100}{1 + \exp\left(\theta_2\left(x - \theta_1\right)\right)},$$

and the variance function is

$$\mathrm{Var}(\varepsilon_i) = \sigma^2(1 + \tau_1 f(x_i, \theta)(100 + \tau_2 - f(x_i, \theta))). \tag{4.6}$$

Method The parameters are estimated by maximizing the log-likelihood, $V(\theta, \sigma^2, \tau)$; see Equation (3.8).

Results We start the estimation process, using for initial parameter values, the estimations of θ and τ_1 calculated with the model defined by Equations (4.2) and (4.3) and $\tau_2 = 0$. We find the following results after 500 iterations of the iterative process:

	Initial Values	Estimated Values	Estimated Standard Error
θ_1	43.93	44.65	0.430
θ_2	0.433	0.778	0.0393
τ_1	0.024	300898	106278
τ_2	0	0.138	0.0061

The estimation process did not converge because the variations of the likelihood are very slow, even for very big variations of τ_1. Figure 4.17 shows the variations of V versus the parameter values obtained at iterations $250, 255, \ldots 500$. It appears that when τ_1 varies from 17,000 to 270,000, V varies from -247.8 to -247.3.

Let us try to run the estimation process with another model for the variance function defined as follows:

$$\sigma_i^2 = \sigma^2 \exp\left(\tau_1 f(x_i, \theta)(100 + \tau_2 - f(x_i, \theta))\right) = g\left(x_i, \theta, \sigma^2, \tau_1, \tau_2\right).$$

This function is obviously different from the preceding polynomial variance function, but the curve is concave and looks like a bell-shaped curve. Moreover, it is often preferable to model a variance function as a function of the exponential function because the result is always positive. Let us see the results with this new model.

Model The regression function is

$$f(x, \theta) = \frac{100}{1 + \exp\left(\theta_2\left(x - \theta_1\right)\right)},$$

and the variance function is

$$\mathrm{Var}(\varepsilon_i) = \sigma^2 \exp\left(\tau_1 f(x_i, \theta)(100 + \tau_2 - f(x_i, \theta))\right). \tag{4.7}$$

Method The parameters are estimated by maximizing the log-likelihood, $V(\theta, \sigma^2, \tau)$; see Equation (3.8).

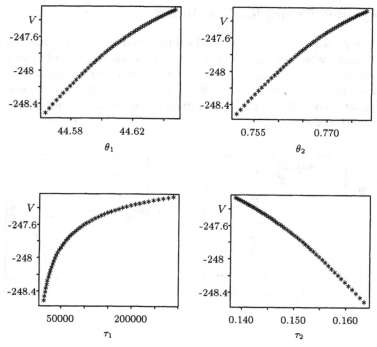

Figure 4.17. Peptides example: Variations of the likelihood against the parameters' values during the estimation process. For each parameter to be estimated, the values of the parameter at iterations $250, 255, \ldots 500$ are reported on the horizontal axis, the corresponding values of the log-likelihood are reported on the vertical axis

Results We start the estimation process using, for initial parameter values, the estimations of θ calculated with the model defined by Equations (4.2) and (4.3) and $\tau_2 = 0$. To choose the initial value for τ_1, we compare the maximum in f of the function $\exp(\tau_1 f(100 - f))$, equal to $\exp 50^2 \tau_1$, to the maximum of the function $1 + \tau_1 f(100 - f)$, equal to $1 + 50^2 \tau_1$. Thus $\tau_1 = 50^{-2} \log(1 + 50^2 \times 0.024)$ is a possible initial value for τ_1. We take $\tau_1 = 0.001$.

	Initial Values	Estimated Values	Estimated Standard Error
θ_1	43.93	45.07	0.422
θ_2	0.433	0.327	0.0223
τ_1	0.001	0.0025	0.00018
τ_2	0	10.45	1.41
σ^2		2.766	

After 49 iterations, the estimation process did converge. Thus, in this particular case we were able to circumvent the numerical difficulty using another variance function. The shape of this function is nearly similar to the shape of the initial variance function defined by Equation (4.6). Let us conclude this chapter by pursuing the discussion about the peptides example.

4.5 Peptides Example: Concluded

Figure 4.18 presents the graph of fitted values, residuals, and standardized absolute residuals when we use the exponential function to model the variations of the variance. Figures 4.18(a) and (b) show that the response is overestimated on its set of variation. Looking at Figure 4.18(c), it appears that the absolute standardized residuals versus fitted values do not present any particular structure.

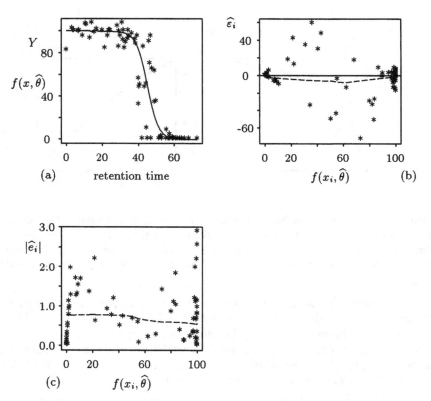

Figure 4.18. Peptides example: Graphs of fitted values and residuals using the exponential variance function: (a) observed and fitted values of the solubility versus the retention time; (b) residuals versus fitted values, the solid line is the horizontal line passing through 0, and the dotted line is a curve joining the points after smoothing; and (c) absolute standardized residuals versus fitted values, the dotted line is a curve joining the points after smoothing

Obviously, we cannot be satisfied with a bad estimation of the response curve. This poor fit is due to the choice of variance function. Using model (4.7) has two effects. The first is, as expected, to take into account the bigger variability of the data when the peptide is fully soluble than when it is nonsoluble.

With model (4.3), the fitted variance when $f = 0$ or $f = 100$ equals $\widehat{\sigma}^2 = 26.79$ (see the results given in Section 4.2.3). With model (4.7), the fitted variance when $f = 0$ is $\widehat{\sigma}^2 = 2.77$, while it is $\widehat{\sigma}^2 \exp(100\widehat{\tau}_1\widehat{\tau}_2) = 38.9$ when $f = 100$. The second effect is to increase considerably the fitted variances when the response lies between 30 and 70, as shown in Figure 4.19. Thus, the weights allowed for observations obtained for values of retention times between 40 and 50 are very low relative to the weights given for observations obtained for values of retention times close to 0 and 60. This explains the overestimation of the response.

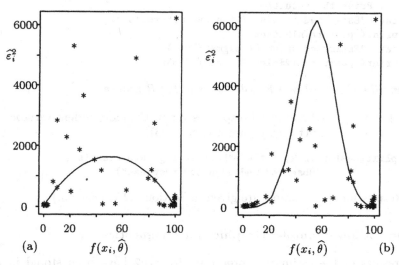

Figure 4.19. Peptides example: Squared residuals $\widehat{\varepsilon}_i^2$ versus adjusted regression function $f(x_i, \widehat{\theta})$. The superimposed lines represent the fitted variances $g(x_i, \widehat{\theta}, \widehat{\sigma}^2, \widehat{\tau})$ versus the $f(x_i, \widehat{\theta})$: (a) variance function (4.3); and (b) (4.7).

4.6 Using nls2

This section reproduces the commands and files used in this chapter to analyze the examples using **nls2**.

Pasture Regrowth Example: Parameter Estimation and Plotting the Observed and Fitted Values of the Response

Parameter Estimation

In a file called **pasture.mod2**, we describe the model defined by Equation (4.1) in Section 4.2.1, page 95:

```
resp yield;
varind time;
parresp p1, p2, p3;
subroutine;
begin
yield=(p2 + p1*time)/(time+p3);
end
```

The parameters are estimated using the function nls2:

```
> pasture.nl2<-nls2(pasture,"pasture.mod2",c(70,-2,20))
>   # Print the results
> cat( "Estimated values of the parameters:\n ")
> print( pasture.nl2$theta)
> cat( "Estimated value of sigma2:\n ")
> print( pasture.nl2$sigma2); cat( "\n\n")
```

Plotting the Observed and Fitted Values of the Response

To plot the observed and fitted responses versus the independent variable, we use the function plfit (see Figure 4.1, page 96):

```
> plfit(pasture.nl2, title ="Pasture regrowth example",
        sub = "Observed and adjusted response")
```

(Results for this example are given in Section 4.2.1, page 95.)

Isomerization Example: Graphics for Diagnostics

The results of the estimation procedure by nls2 have been stored in the structure called isomer.nl1 (see Section 1.6, page 26).

Plotting the Fitted Values of the Response Against Its Observed Values

To plot the fitted values of the response against its observed values, we use the function plfit:

- Option smooth means that the observed values are joined after smoothing.
- Option wanted specifies the graph requested, fitted values versus observed values of the response.
- Option ask.modify allows us to type an S-Plus command before the graph disappears from the screen. Here, we type the abline command to add the first diagonal on the plot:

```
> plfit(isomer.nl1, smooth=T, wanted=list(O.F=T),
        title="Isomerization example",
        ask.modify=T)
> abline(0,1)
```

(See Figure 4.2, page 96.)

Plotting the Residuals

The function **plres** is used to plot the residuals.

Option **wanted** specifies the graphs requested. Its values are:

- **F.R**: The residuals are plotted against the fitted values of the response.
- **R.R**: The residuals are plotted against the immediately preceding residuals.
- **I.R**: The residuals are plotted against their indexes.

Option **absolute** means that the absolute values of the residuals are added on the graphs corresponding to **F.R** and **I.R**:

```
> plres(isomer.nl1,
      wanted=list(F.R=T, R.R=T, I.R=T),
      absolute=T,
      title="Isomerization example")
```

(See Figure 4.3, page 97.)

Solubility of Peptides Example: Graphics for Diagnostics

Plotting the Observed and Fitted Values of the Response When Variance is Assumed to be Constant

The results of estimation with the model defined in Section 3.1.2 (logistic curve for the regression function and constant variances) have been stored in the structure **pept.nl1** (see Section 3.6, page 89). Now we plot the observed and fitted responses versus the retention time using the function **plfit**. Option **wanted** specifies the graph requested. The observed and fitted values of the response are plotted against the independent variable:

```
> plfit(pept.nl1, wanted=list(X.OF=T),
        title="Solubility of peptides example - constant variance",
        sub="Observed and fitted response")
```

(See Figure 4.4(a), page 99.)

Plotting the Residuals When Variance is Assumed to be Constant

Residuals and absolute residuals are plotted against the fitted values of the response by using the function **plres**:

- Option **wanted** specifies the graph requested; the fitted values of the residuals are plotted against the fitted values of the response.
- Option **absolute** means that the absolute residuals are plotted.
- Option **smooth** means that the observed values are joined after smoothing.
- Option **ask.modify** allows us to type an S-Plus command before the graph disappears from the screen. Here, we type the **abline** command to add a horizontal line on the plot:

```
> plres.nls2(pept.nl1, wanted=list(F.R=T),
        absolute=T, smooth=T, ask.modify=T,
        title="Solubility of peptides example - constant variance")
> abline(0,0)
```

(See Figures 4.4(b) and (c), page 99.)

Plotting the Observed and Fitted Values of the Response and the Residuals When Variance is Assumed to be Heteroscedastic

In the same way, we draw plots from the structure pept.nl3, which contains the results of estimation when the variance is assumed to be heteroscedastic (see Section 3.6, page 89, and Equation (3.3), page 65).

```
>     # Plot the observed and fitted values of the response
>     # against the independent variable.
> plfit(pept.nl3, wanted=list(X.OF=T),
        title="Solubility of peptides - non constant variance",
        sub="Observed and fitted response")
>     # Plot the residuals
> plres.nls2(pept.nl3, wanted=list(F.R=T),
        absolute=T, st=T, smooth=T, ask.modify=T,
        title="Solubility of peptides - non constant variance")
> abline(0,0)
```

(See Figure 4.5, page 100.)

Cortisol Assay Example: How to Choose the Variance Function Using Replications

Estimation Using a Symmetric Sigmoidally Shaped Regression Curve and a Constant Variance

We first estimate the parameters using the model defined in Section 4.2.4, page 99 (symmetric regression curve and constant variance). When the parameter θ_5 is equal to 1, this model is similar to the model we described in the file corti.mod1 (asymmetric regression curve and constant variance; see Section 1.6, page 21). So, by setting a numerical equality constraint on the fifth parameter, we can reuse the file corti.mod1 when calling nls2:

```
> corti.nl3<-nls2(corti,
    list(file="corti.mod1",gamf=c(0,10), eq.theta=c(rep(NaN,4),1)),
    c(corti.nl1$theta[1:4],1))
>     # Print the main results
> cat( "Estimated values of the parameters:\n ")
> print(coef(corti.nl3))
> cat( "Estimated value of sigma2:\n ")
> print( corti.nl3$sigma2); cat( "\n\n")
```

Plotting the Response Values and the Residuals When the Regression Function is a Symmetric Sigmoidally Shaped Curve and the Variance is Constant

We use the graphical functions of S-Plus to plot the observed and fitted values of the response versus the log-dose. The observed values are joined by a line. Then we plot the residuals and absolute residuals versus the fitted values of the response using the function `plres`:

```
>      # Plot the observed and fitted values of the response
>      # against the log-dose
> plot(logdose,corti$cpm,xlab="log-dose",ylab="response")
> title(main="Cortisol example",
          sub="Observed and adjusted response")
> lines(unique(logdose),corti.nl3$response)
>      # Plot the residuals
> plres(corti.nl3,
          wanted=list(F.R=T),
          absolute=T,
          title="Cortisol example")
```

(See Figure 4.6, page 101.)

Plotting the Empirical Variances Versus the Empirical Means When the Regression Function is a Symmetric Sigmoidally Shaped Curve and the Variance is Constant

To plot the variances, we use the graphical function `plvar`. This function offers many choices. Using option **wanted**, we specify the graphs requested:

- Y.S2 to plot the empirical variances against the empirical means,
- Y.S to plot the square roots of the empirical variances against the empirical means, and
- logY.logS2 to plot the logarithms of the empirical variances against the logarithms of the means.

Option smooth means that the observed values are joined after smoothing:

```
> plvar(corti.nl3,wanted=list(Y.S2=T,Y.S=T,logY.logS2=T),
    smooth=T,
    title="Cortisol example")
```

(See Figure 4.7, page 102.)

Estimation Using a Symmetric Sigmoidally Shaped Regression Curve and a Heteroscedastic Variance

Now we study the model defined in Equation (4.4), page 102 (symmetric sigmoidal regression curve and heteroscedastic variances).

We describe it in a file called `corti.mod6`. Actually, `corti.mod6` corresponds to an asymmetric model but, by setting the fifth parameter `g` to 1, it is equivalent to a symmetric one. By doing so, we will not have to create another file when we study the asymmetric model:

```
% model CORTI
resp cpm;
var v;
varind dose;
parresp n,d,a,b,g;
pbisresp minf,pinf;
subroutine;
begin
cpm= if dose <= minf then d else
        if dose >= pinf then n else
        n+(d-n)*exp(-g*log(1+exp(a+b*log10(dose))))
    fi fi;
v = cpm**2;
end
```

We estimate the parameters using `nls2`, remembering to set a numerical constraint on the last parameter:

```
> corti.nl6<-nls2(corti,
    list(file= "corti.mod6",gamf=c(0,10), eq.theta=c(rep(NaN,4),1)),
    c(corti.nl1$theta[1:4],1))
>      # Print the main results
> cat( "Estimated values of the parameters:\n ")
> print(coef(corti.nl6))
> cat( "Estimated value of sigma2:\n ")
> print( corti.nl6$sigma2); cat( "\n\n")
```

Plotting the Observed and Fitted Values of the Response and the Residuals When the Regression Function is a Symmetric Sigmoidally Shaped Curve and the Variance is Heteroscedastic

We plot the observed and fitted values of the response using graphical functions of S-Plus and the residuals using the function `plres`:

```
>      # Plot the observed and fitted values of the response
>      # against the log-dose
> plot(logdose,corti$cpm,xlab="log-dose",ylab="response")
> title(main="Cortisol example",
        sub="Observed and adjusted response")
> lines(unique(logdose),corti.nl6$response)
>      # Plot the residuals
> plres(corti.nl6,
        wanted=list(F.R=T),
        absolute=T,st=T,smooth=T,
        title="Cortisol example",ask.modify=T)
> abline(0,0)
```

(See Figure 4.8, page 104.)

Estimation Using an Asymmetric Sigmoidally Shaped Regression Curve and a Heteroscedastic Variance

Finally, we study the last model defined in Equation (4.5), page 103 (asymmetric sigmoidal regression curve and heteroscedastic variances). It is similar to the previous one, where we suppress the constraint on the last parameter. So, when calling nls2, we reuse the file corti.mod6:

```
> corti.nl7<-nls2(corti,
      list(file="corti.mod6",gamf=c(0,10)),
      corti.nl6$theta)
>      # Print the main results
> cat( "Estimated values of the parameters:\n ")
> print(coef(corti.nl7))
> cat( "Estimated value of sigma2:\n ")
> print( corti.nl7$sigma2); cat( "\n\n")
```

Plotting the Observed and Fitted Values of the Response and the Residuals When the Regression Function is an Asymmetric Sigmoidally Shaped Curve and the Variance is Heteroscedastic

We plot the observed and fitted values of the response and the residuals:

```
>      # Plot the observed and fitted values of the response
>      # against the log-dose
> plot(logdose,corti$cpm,xlab="log-dose",ylab="response")
> title(main="Cortisol example",
        sub="Observed and adjusted response")
> lines(unique(logdose),corti.nl7$response)
> plres(corti.nl7,
        wanted=list(F.R=T),
        absolute=T,st=T,smooth=T,
        title="Cortisol example",ask.modify=T)
> abline(0,0)
```

(See Figure 4.9, page 105.)

Trajectory of Roots of Maize: How to Detect Correlations in Errors

This is a new example, introduced in this chapter. We first create a *data frame* to store the experimental data. Then we plot the observed values of the response against the independent variable.

Creating the Data

Experimental data are stored in a *data frame* called root:

```
> root_data.frame(depth = c(0, 0.687, 1.523, 1.981, 2.479,
        3.535, 4.46, 5.506, 6.582, 7.519, 8.615, 9.591,
        10.588, 11.604, 12.471, 13.507,
        14.534, 15.45, 16.496, 17.443, 18.5, 19.516, 20.603,
        21.53, 22.547, 23.514, 24.51, 25.606, 26.503, 27.579,
        28.476, 29.512, 30.569, 31.675, 32.613, 33.539, 34.626,
        35.563, 36.599, 37.636, 38.712, 40.068, 40.657,
        41.445, 41.983, 42.94, 43.897, 44.934, 45.941, 46.948,
        47.935, 48.982, 50.049, 50.996, 51.913, 52.95, 53.887,
        54.904, 56.021, 57.028, 57.975, 59.002, 59.979, 61.046,
        61.963, 63.079, 63.937, 65.113, 66.18, 66.958,
        67.965, 68.942, 70.098, 70.985, 71.952, 72.849, 74.165,
        75.082, 75.88, 77.007, 78.054, 78.174, 79.091, 80.128,
        81.035, 82.032, 83.019, 84.185, 85.042, 86.089, 87.156,
        88.023, 89.15, 89.997, 91.124, 92.829),
        dist =
        c(-0.009, 3.012, 6.064, 8.726, 10.102, 12.166, 19.076,
        21.967, 23.882, 25.916, 27.143, 28.997, 31.101, 32.667,
        34.691, 36.227, 37.643, 39.827, 41.951, 43.227, 44.105,
        44.584, 45.053, 45.691, 46.25, 47.038, 49.561, 51.077,
        52.523, 55.005, 55.833, 56.432, 57.1, 57.749, 58.178,
        58.966, 59.823, 61.708, 62.476, 62.945, 63.873, 63.763,
        63.789, 63.889, 64.188, 64.348, 64.598, 64.628, 64.638,
        64.678, 64.559, 64.47, 64.4, 64.271, 64.042, 63.943,
        63.873, 63.844, 63.983, 64.253, 64.323, 64.333, 64.354,
        64.643, 64.933, 65.122, 65.222, 65.372, 65.522, 65.523,
        65.523, 65.533, 65.932, 66.361, 66.691, 67.04, 67.459,
        67.549, 67.579, 67.59, 67.161, 65.825, 65.477, 65.886,
        66.415, 66.844, 67.233, 67.901, 67.911, 68.251,
        68.251, 68.241, 68.621, 68.92, 68.92, 68.383))
```

Plotting the Observed Responses Against the Independent Variable

To plot the observed responses versus the depth in the ground, we use the graphical function pldnls2:

```
> pldnls2(root,response.name="dist",X.names="depth")
```

(See Figure 4.10, page 106.)

Parameter Estimation

We describe the next model defined in Section 4.2.5, page 104 in a file called root.mod1:

```
resp dist;
varind depth;
parresp b,g;
subroutine;
begin
dist=b*(1-exp(-g*depth));
end
```

To estimate the parameters, we use the function **nls2**:

```
> root.nl1<-nls2(root,"root.mod1",c(70,1))
>      # Print the estimated values
> cat( "Estimated values of the parameters:\n ")
> print(root.nl1$theta); cat( "\n\n")
```

Plotting the Observed and Fitted Values of the Response and the Residuals

We plot the observed and fitted responses versus the depth in the ground using the function **plfit**. Option **wanted** specifies the graph requested: **X.OF** means that observed and fitted values are plotted against the independent variable. Then we plot the residuals using the function **plres**. Here, with option **wanted**, we ask for the plot of the residuals versus the preceding residual (see Figure 4.11, page 106):

```
>      # Plot the observed and fitted values of the response
>      # against the independent variable.
> plfit(root.nl1,
          wanted=list(X.OF=T),
          title="Trajectory of roots")
>      # Plot the residuals
> plres(root.nl1,
          wanted=list(R.R=T),
          title="Trajectory of roots")
```

(Results for this example are given in Section 4.2.5, page 103.)

Simulated Example

Creating the First Data Set

The way data are generated is fully explained in Section 4.2.6, page 107.

To generate the 10 values of ε_i, $i = 1, \ldots 10$, we use the S-Plus function **rnorm** (random generation for the normal distribution, with given values of means and standard deviations):

```
# x1<-seq(0.1,1.,length=10)
# exserr<-rnorm(10, mean=0, sd=.05)
# exsw1<-data.frame(x=x1,
#                   y=1-exp(-x1)+exserr)
```

Actually, we do not execute these commands because random generation would not create the same data as shown herein. Instead, we create the *data frame* explicitly:

```
> exsw1 <- data.frame(
    x = c(0.1, 0.2, 0.3, 0.4, 0.5, 0.6, 0.7, 0.8, 0.9, 1),
    y = c(0.1913, 0.0737, 0.2702, 0.4270, 0.2968, 0.4474,
             0.4941, 0.5682, 0.5630, 0.6636))
```

Parameter Estimation with the First Data Set

We describe the model defined in Section 4.2.6, page 107 in a file called sim.mod1:

```
resp y;
varind x;
parresp p1,p2;
subroutine;
begin
y=p1*(1-exp(-p2*x));
end
```

The function nls2 is used to estimate the parameters:

```
> sim.nl1<-nls2(exsw1,"sim.mod1",c(1,1))
>    # Print the main results
> cat( "Estimated values of the parameters:\n ")
> print(coef(sim.nl1))
> cat( "Estimated value of sigma2:\n ")
> print(sim.nl1$sigma2); cat( "\n\n")
```

We calculate the confidence intervals for the parameters:

```
> confsim <- confidence(sim.nl1)
> cat( "Confidence interval for the parameters:\n")
> print(confsim$normal.conf.int); cat( "\n\n")
```

Plotting the Generated and Fitted Values of the Response with the First Data Set

We plot the generated and fitted values of the response versus x using the function plfit:

```
> plfit(sim.nl1, wanted=list(X.OF=T),title="Simulated example 1")
```

(See Figure 4.12, page 108.)

Plotting Sensitivity Functions for the First Data Set

The sensitivity functions Φ_1 and Φ_2 described herein are calculated in the
nls2.object for the values of x in the data set. We plot their values versus
x:

```
> matplot(exsw1$x, sim.nl1$d.resp,type="l",xlab="x",ylab="")
> legend(x=0.5,y=.3,legend=c("phi1","phi2"),lty=c(1,2))
> title(" Plot of sensitivity functions")
```

(See Figure 4.13, page 109.)

Creating the Second Data Set

Another data set is generated with more appropriate values of x:

```
# exsw2 <- data.frame(x=seq(0.1,4.6,length=10),
#                        y=1-exp(-x2)+exserr)
```

To consider the same data as shown earlier (see page 108), we do not
execute these commands but type the values explicitly:

```
> exsw2  <-  data.frame(
       x = c(0.1, 0.6, 1.1, 1.6, 2.1, 2.6, 3.1, 3.6, 4.1, 4.6),
       y = c(0.1913, 0.3436, 0.6782, 0.8954, 0.7809, 0.9220,
              0.9457, 0.9902, 0.9530, 1.0215))
```

Parameter Estimation with the Second Data Set

The parameters are estimated using nls2:

```
>   sim.nl2 <- nls2(exsw2,"sim.mod1",c(1,1))
>    # Print the main results
> cat( "Estimated values of the parameters:\n ")
> print(coef(sim.nl2))
```

*Plotting the Generated and Fitted Values of the Response with the Second
Data Set*

We plot the generated and fitted values of the responses versus x using the
function plfit (see Figure 4.14, page 110):

```
> plfit(sim.nl2,
         wanted=list(X.OF=T),
         title="Simulated example 2")
```

(Results for this example are given in Section 4.2.6, page 107.)

Cortisol Assay Example: Misspecification Tests

Comparison of Nested Models

The test of hypothesis H against the alternative A defined on page 110 is done by calculating the difference of the log-likelihoods stored in `corti.nl6` and `corti.nl7`. We compare it to the 0.95 quantile of a χ^2 with one degree of freedom (see Section 4.3.1, page 110):

```
> Sl <- 64*(corti.nl6$loglik - corti.nl7$loglik)
> cat( "Sl: ", Sl,  "X2(0.95,1): ",qchisq(0.95,1),"\n ")
```

Test When the Regression Function is Symmetric and the Variance Proportional to the Squared Expectation

The results of estimation with the first model, H, defined in Section 4.3.3, page 112 (the regression function is symmetric and the variance proportional to the squared expectation), have been stored in the structure called `corti.nl6` (see page 123).

We test the model H against the alternative A_2 (homogeneous variance) by calculating the test statistic S_L. We compare it to the 0.95 quantile of a χ^2 with 25 degrees of freedom (see Section 4.3.2, page 110):

```
> Sl <- sum(corti.nl6$replications*log(corti.nl6$variance))-
        sum(corti.nl6$replications*log(corti.nl6$data.stat$S2))
> k <- length(corti.nl6$replications) # number of observations
> cat( "Sl:", Sl,
    "\nX2(0.95,25):",qchisq(0.95, 2*k - 5),"\n\n"  )
```

Test When the Regression Function is an Asymmetric Sigmoidally Shaped Curve and the Variance Heteroscedastic

The results of the estimation when the regression function is an asymmetric sigmoidally shaped curve and the variance heteroscedastic (the second model defined in Section 4.3.3, page 112) have been stored in the structure `corti.nl7` (see page 125).

We calculate the test statistic S_L and compare it to the 0.95 quantile of a χ^2 with 24 degrees of freedom:

```
> Sl <- sum(corti.nl7$replications*log(corti.nl7$variance))-
        sum(corti.nl7$replications*log(corti.nl7$data.stat$S2))
> cat( "Sl:", Sl,
    "\nX2(0.95,24):",qchisq(0.95, 2*k - 6),"\n\n"  )
```

(Results for this example are given in Section 4.3.3, page 112.)

Ovocytes Example: Graphic and Misspecification Tests Using Replications

The results of the estimation for the model defined in Section 4.3.4 page 112, have been stored in the structure `ovo.nl1` (see page 25).

Plotting the Residuals and the Variances

We use the function `plres` to plot the residuals and the absolute residuals versus the fitted values of the response and the function `plvar` to plot the empirical variances versus the empirical means:

```
>     # Plot the residuals
> plres(ovo.nl1, wanted=list(F.R=T), absolute=T,
         title="Ovocytes example")
>     # Plot the variances
> plvar(ovo.nl1,wanted=list(Y.S2=T),smooth=T,
         title="Ovocytes example")
```

(See Figure 4.15, page 113, and Figure 4.16, page 114.)

Test

We calculate the test statistic S_L and compare it to the 0.95 quantile of a χ^2 with 53 degrees of freedom:

```
> n <- sum(ovo.nl1$replications) # total number of replications
> k <- length(ovo.nl1$replications) # number of observations
> Sl <- n*log(ovo.nl1$sigma2) -
         sum(ovo.nl1$replications*log(ovo.nl1$data.stat$S2))
> cat( "Sl:", Sl,
    "\nX2(0.95,53):",qchisq(0.95, 2*k - 5),"\n\n"  )
```

(Results for this example are given in Section 4.3.4, page 112.)

Solubility of Peptides Example: Numerical Troubles During the Estimation Process

Estimation with the Model Defined by Equation (4.6)

The model defined by Equation (4.6) is described in a file called `pept.m13`:

```
% model pept.m13
resp solubility;
varind RetTime;
var v;
aux a1;
parresp ed50, sl ;
parvar h1, h2;
subroutine ;
begin
a1 = 1 + exp (sl*(RetTime-ed50)) ;
solubility = 100. /a1 ;
v= 1 + h1*solubility*(100+h2-solubility);
end
```

We estimate the parameters with this model. Here, to be able to draw Figure 4.17, page 117 (variations of V versus the parameter values at iterations $250, 255, \ldots 500$), we must request that the results calculated thorough the iterative process be saved. With the `control` argument, we request that the estimated values of the parameters and the statistical criterion are saved after every five iterations. Using the option `wanted.print`, we suppress the printing of intermediary results:

```
> pept.ctx13<-list(theta.start=pept.nl3$theta,
            beta.start=c(pept.nl3$beta,0),max.iters=500)
> pept.ctr13<-list(
        freq=5,step.iters.sv=1,
        wanted.iters.sv=list(iter=T,estim=T,stat.crit=T),
        wanted.print=list(iter=F,stat.crit=F,stop.crit=F,
                    estim=F,fitted=F,num.res=F,sigma2=F))
> pept.nl13<-nls2(pept.d, "pept.m13", pept.ctx13,control=pept.ctr13)
> # Print the result
> summary(pept.nl13)
```

The intermediary results are saved in the component `iters.sv` of the returned structure. The last 50 elements contain the results obtained at iterations $250, 255, \ldots, 500$. So we can draw Figure 4.17, page 117, using the following commands:

```
> ind<-50:100
> par(mfrow=c(2,2))
> plot(pept.nl13$iters.sv$theta[ind,1],
    -75*pept.nl13$iters.sv$stat.crit[ind]/2)
> plot(pept.nl13$iters.sv$theta[ind,2],
    -75*pept.nl13$iters.sv$stat.crit[ind]/2)
> plot(pept.nl13$iters.sv$beta[ind,1],
    -75*pept.nl13$iters.sv$stat.crit[ind]/2)
> plot(pept.nl13$iters.sv$beta[ind,2],
    -75*pept.nl13$iters.sv$stat.crit[ind]/2)
```

Estimation with the Model Defined by Equation (4.7)

The model defined by Equation (4.7) is described in a file called `pept.m14`:

```
% model pept.m14
resp solubility;
varind RetTime;
var v;
aux a1;
parresp ed50, sl ;
parvar h1, h2;
subroutine ;
begin
a1 = 1 + exp (sl*(RetTime-ed50)) ;
solubility = 100. /a1 ;
```

```
v= exp(h1*solubility*(100+h2-solubility)));
end
```

We estimate the parameters with this model:

```
> pept.ctx14<-list(theta.start=pept.nl3$theta,
                   beta.start=c(0.001,0),max.iters=500)
> pept.nl14<-nls2(pept.d, "pept.m14", pept.ctx14)
> # Print the result
> summary(pept.nl14)
```

Peptides Example: Concluded

We draw plots from the structure `pept.nl14` (see Figure 4.18, page 118):

```
>      # Plot the observed and fitted values of the response
>      # against the independent variable.
> plfit(pept.nl14, wanted=list(X.OF=T),
       title="Solubility of peptides - exponential variance",
       sub="Observed and fitted response")
>      # Plot the residuals
> plres.nls2(pept.nl14, wanted=list(F.R=T),
       smooth=T, ask.modify=T,
       title="Solubility of peptides - exponential variance")
> abline(0,0)
> plres.nls2(pept.nl14, wanted=list(F.R=T),
       absolute=T, st=T, smooth=T, ask.modify=T,
       title="Solubility of peptides - exponential variance")
```

For both models, we plot the squared residuals versus the fitted values of the regression function. We add a line to join the fitted values of the variances:

```
> par(mfrow=c(1,2))
> plot(range(pept.nl14$response),
     range(c(pept.nl14$residuals**2,pept.nl14$variance)),
     xlab="fitted responses", ylab="squared residuals")
> title(main="Parabolic variance function")
> points(rep(pept.nl3$response,pept.nl3$replications),
     pept.nl3$residuals**2)
> lines(sort(pept.nl3$response),
     pept.nl3$variance[order(pept.nl3$response)],lty=1)
> plot(range(pept.nl14$response),
     range(c(pept.nl14$residuals**2,pept.nl14$variance)),
     xlab="fitted responses", ylab="squared residuals")
> title(main="Exponential variance function")
> points(rep(pept.nl14$response,pept.nl14$replications),
     pept.nl14$residuals**2)
> lines(sort(pept.nl14$response),
     pept.nl14$variance[order(pept.nl14$response)],lty=1)
```

(See Figure 4.19, page 119.)

5

Calibration and Prediction

In this chapter, we describe how to calculate *prediction* and calibration confidence intervals. These intervals account for the double source of variability that exists in this type of experiment: The variability of the response about its mean and the uncertainty about the regression parameters. Here we provide both bootstrap and asymptotic methods for the prediction and calibration confidence intervals.

5.1 Examples

To illustrate the prediction problem, let us recall the pasture regrowth example and assume that we are interested in predicting the yield y_0 at the time $x_0 = 50$. We wish to obtain point and interval predictors for the response y_0, which has not been observed.

In Example 1.1.2, we estimated the calibration curve of an RIA of cortisol. The real interest of the assay experiment, however, lies in estimating an unknown dose of hormone contained in a new preparation. For this new preparation, we observe a response y_0, and we want to draw inferences about the true dose x_0 corresponding to the new value y_0 of the count. This is a typical calibration problem.

To further illustrate the problem of calibration, let us introduce another example from a bioassay described by Racine-Poon [RP88].

Bioassay on Nasturtium

The objective of this experiment is to determine the concentrations of an agrochemical present in soil samples. To this end, bioassays are performed on test plants, a type of cress called *nasturtium*.

In a first step, called the calibration experiment, six replicates Y_{ij} of the response are measured at seven predetermined concentrations x_i of the soil sample.

Table 5.1. Data from the calibration experiment on nasturtium

Concentration (g/ha)	Weight (mg)					
0.000	920	889	866	930	992	1017
0.025	919	878	882	854	851	850
0.075	870	825	953	834	810	875
0.250	880	834	795	837	834	810
0.750	693	690	722	738	563	591
2.000	429	395	435	412	273	257
4.000	200	244	209	225	128	221

Table 5.2. Observed weights corresponding to new soil samples from the field

New Experiment	Weight (mg)		
x_0?	309	296	419

The response is the weight of the plant after three weeks' growth, as shown in Table 5.1.

In a second step, three replicates of the response at an unknown concentration of interest x_0 are measured; they are listed in Table 5.2. We would like to estimate x_0.

Figure 5.1 shows the responses observed in the calibration experiment as a function of the logarithm of the concentration. The 0 concentration is represented in Figure 5.1 by the value -5. A logit-log model is used to describe

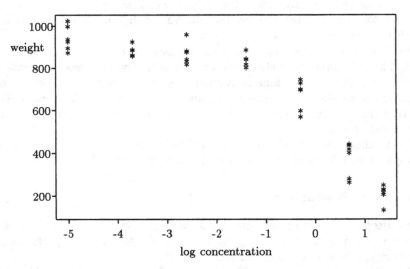

Figure 5.1. Nasturtium example: Weights versus the log concentration

the concentration response relationship:

$$f(x, \theta) = \theta_1 \qquad\qquad\qquad\qquad \text{if } x = 0,$$
$$= \theta_1/(1 + \exp(\theta_2 + \theta_3 \log(x))) \quad \text{if } x > 0,$$

where x is the concentration and $f(x, \theta)$ is the expected weight of nasturtium at concentration x.

The model under study is the following one:

$$\left. \begin{array}{c} Y_{ij} = f(x_i, \theta) + \varepsilon_{ij} \\ \text{Var}(\varepsilon_{ij}) = \sigma^2 \end{array} \right\}, \qquad (5.1)$$

where $j = 1, \ldots 6$; $i = 1, \ldots 7$; and the ε_{ij} are independent centered random variables.

5.2 Problem Formulation

In prediction or calibration experiments, we first observe a training or calibration data set, (x_i, Y_{ij}), $j = 1, \ldots, n_i$, $n = \sum n_i$, from which the response curve (or calibration curve) and the variance structure are fitted. Let $\widehat{\theta}$ be the least squares estimator of θ in the case of homogeneous variances ($\text{Var}(\varepsilon_{ij}) = \sigma^2$), and let it be the maximum likelihood estimator in the case of heterogeneous variances (see Chapter 3).

The real interest lies in the new pair (x_0, y_0). In prediction problems, x_0 is given and we want to predict the associated response y_0. The standard estimate for y_0 is $f(x_0, \widehat{\theta})$. In calibration problems, y_0 is observed but the unknown value x_0 must be estimated. The usual estimate of x_0 is the set of all x values for which $f(x_0, \widehat{\theta}) = y_0$. For f strictly increasing or decreasing, the estimate will be a single value obtained by inverting the regression function: $\widehat{x_0} = f^{-1}(y_0, \widehat{\theta})$.

5.3 Confidence Intervals

5.3.1 Prediction of a Response

Let us begin by discussing the problem of prediction with constant variances, which will provide motivation for the more prevalent problem of calibration.

Given the value x_0, the variance of the error made in predicting y_0 is $\text{Var}(y_0 - f(x_0, \widehat{\theta}))$. If homogeneous variances are assumed, we first obtain $\widehat{\theta}$. Then we estimate σ^2 by the residual sum of squares $\widehat{\sigma}^2$ and the variance of $f(x_0, \widehat{\theta})$ by $\widehat{S}$, as explained in Section 2.3.1. The required *prediction interval* is

$$\widehat{I}_N(x_0) = \left[f(x_0, \widehat{\theta}) - \nu_{1-\alpha/2} \widehat{S}_{\widehat{f}} \,;\, f(x_0, \widehat{\theta}) + \nu_{1-\alpha/2} \widehat{S}_{\widehat{f}} \right], \qquad (5.2)$$

where

$$\widehat{S}_{\widehat{f}}^2 = \widehat{\sigma}^2 + \widehat{S}^2 \tag{5.3}$$

and ν_α is the α percentile of a variate distributed as an $\mathcal{N}(0,1)$. Under the assumption that y_0 is a Gaussian variable, $\widehat{I}_{\mathcal{N}}(x_0)$ has asymptotic level $1 - \alpha$. It is interesting to compare Equation (5.2) with Equation (2.2), taking $\lambda = f(x_0, \theta)$, because Equation (2.2) provides a confidence interval for the mean $f(x_0, \theta)$ rather than for the response itself.

Remark If the size n of the calibration data set is large, the variance term is dominated by $\widehat{\sigma}^2$, signifying that the uncertainty in predicting y_0 is mostly due to its variability about its mean. The second term, $\widehat{S}^2$, is the correction for estimation of θ. However, for moderate n, $\widehat{S}^2$ can be of the same order of magnitude as $\widehat{\sigma}^2$.

Bootstrap Prediction Intervals

The bootstrap method described in Section 2.3.5 replaces the normal percentiles ν_α, $\nu_{1-\alpha/2}$ in Equation (5.2) by bootstrap percentiles using the bootstrap distribution as a better approximation to the distribution of

$$\widehat{T} = \frac{y_0 - f(x_0, \widehat{\theta})}{\left\{\widehat{\sigma}^2 + \widehat{S}^2\right\}^{1/2}}.$$

As a result, we obtain more accurate prediction intervals.

Bootstrap prediction intervals are based on the quantiles of

$$\widehat{T}^\star = \frac{y_0^\star - f(x_0, \widehat{\theta}^\star)}{\left\{\widehat{\sigma}^{2\star} + S_{\widehat{\theta}^\star}^2\right\}^{1/2}},$$

where $\widehat{\theta}^\star$ and $\widehat{\sigma}^{2\star}$ are bootstrap estimations of θ and σ^2 that are calculated from bootstrap samples $(x_i, Y_{ij}^\star)$, $j = 1, \ldots, n_i$, $i = 1, \ldots, k$, where

$$Y_{ij}^\star = f(x_i, \widehat{\theta}) + \varepsilon_{ij}^\star$$

and

$$y_0^\star = f(x_0, \widehat{\theta}) + \varepsilon_0^\star$$

is the "new" bootstrap observation. Here $(\varepsilon_{ij}^\star, \varepsilon_0^\star)$ is an independent bootstrap sample of the errors of length $n + 1$. The method of generating the errors $\varepsilon_{ij}^\star$ and $\varepsilon_0^\star$ from the residuals $\widehat{\varepsilon}_{ij} = Y_{ij} - f(x_i, \widehat{\theta})$ was detailed in Section 2.3.5.

Let B be the number of bootstrap simulations. $(\widehat{T}^{\star,b}, b = 1, \ldots B)$ is a B sample of $\widehat{T}^\star$. Let b_α be the α percentile of the $\widehat{T}^{\star,b}$ (the method of calculating b_α was detailed in Section 2.4.1). This gives a bootstrap prediction interval for y_0 of the following form:

$$\widehat{I}_B(x_0) = \left[f(x_0, \widehat{\theta}) - b_{1-\alpha/2} \widehat{S}_{\widehat{f}} \; ; f(x_0, \widehat{\theta}) - b_{\alpha/2} \widehat{S}_{\widehat{f}} \right], \tag{5.4}$$

where $\widehat{S}_{\widehat{f}}$ is defined by Equation (5.3).

For large n and B the coverage probability of $\widehat{I}_B(x_0)$ is close to $1 - \alpha$. In practice, however, a value of B around 200 usually suffices.

Case of Heteroscedastic Variance

When the model under study is defined by Equation (3.7), then the preceding results apply after slight modifications: The estimated variance of $y_0 - f(x_0, \widehat{\theta})$ is $\widehat{S}_{\widehat{f}}^2 = \widehat{\sigma}^2 g(x_0, \widehat{\theta}, \widehat{\tau}) + \widehat{S}^2$, and the resampling scheme used for the bootstrap method is described in Section 3.4.3.

5.3.2 Calibration with Constant Variances

To do a calibration procedure, suppose that we observe m replicates y_{0l}, $l = 1, \ldots, m$, of the response at an unknown x_0 and that we wish to obtain a calibration interval for x_0. Let $\overline{y_0} = \sum_{l=1}^{m} y_{0l}/m$. We suppose that

$$\mathrm{Var}(y_{0l}) = \sigma^2 = \mathrm{Var}(Y_{ij}).$$

A *calibration interval* can be constructed for x_0 by inverting Equation (5.2). In other words, the confidence interval is the set of all x such that $\overline{y_0}$ falls in the corresponding prediction interval $\widehat{I}(x_0)$. A calibration interval for x_0, then, is

$$\widehat{J}_{\mathcal{N}} = \left\{ x, \quad |\overline{y_0} - f(x, \widehat{\theta})| \leq \nu_{1-\alpha/2} \left\{ \frac{\widehat{\sigma}^2}{m} + \widehat{S}^2 \right\}^{1/2} \right\}, \tag{5.5}$$

where $\widehat{S}^2$ is the estimation of the asymptotic variance of $f(x_0, \widehat{\theta})$ calculated at $\widehat{x}_0$.

Like the confidence intervals constructed in Section 2.3.2, $\widehat{J}_{\mathcal{N}}$ has asymptotic level $1 - \alpha$: Its coverage probability should be close to $1 - \alpha$ when both the number of replications m and the size of the calibration data set n tend to infinity. From our experience, however, $\widehat{J}_{\mathcal{N}}$ may have a covering probability significantly different from the expected asymptotic level when n and m have small values.

Bootstrap Calibration Intervals

Using the bootstrap method presented in Section 2.3.5, we can construct *calibration intervals* that actually achieve the desired nominal level, even in small-sample situations.

The construction of bootstrap calibration intervals is based on the simulation of bootstrap samples of the training data (x_i, Y_{ij}^*), $j = 1, \ldots, n_i$, $i = 1, \ldots k$, and on bootstrap samples y_{0l}^* of the responses at x_0. The bootstrap procedure is as follows:

- Let $\tilde{\varepsilon}_{ij}$ be the n centered residuals:

$$\tilde{\varepsilon}_{ij} = Y_{ij} - f(x_i, \widehat{\theta}) - n^{-1} \sum_{i,j} \left(Y_{ij} - f(x_i, \widehat{\theta}) \right),$$

  $j = 1, \ldots, n_i$, $i = 1, \ldots k$. n bootstrap errors ε_{ij}^* are drawn with replacement from the $\tilde{\varepsilon}_{ij}$, each with probability $1/n$. Then $Y_{ij}^* = f(x_i, \widehat{\theta}) + \varepsilon_{ij}^*$. Let $\widehat{\theta}^*$ and $\widehat{\sigma}^{2*}$ denote the bootstrap estimates obtained from the bootstrap sample (x_i, Y_{ij}^*).
- To resample the responses y_{0l}, $l = 1, \ldots, m$, randomly choose m additional bootstrap errors e_l^* from the $\tilde{\varepsilon}_{ij}$ and compute the bootstrap responses at x_0 as $y_{0l}^* = \overline{y_0} + e_l^*$ $l = 1, \ldots, m$. Let $\overline{y_0}^* = \sum_1^m y_{0l}^*/m$.

The resampling scheme can be repeated B times. At each run, we compute

$$\widehat{T}^* = \frac{\overline{y_0}^* - f(\widehat{x_0}, \widehat{\theta}^*)}{\left\{ \frac{1}{m} \widehat{\sigma}^{2*} + \widehat{S}^{2*} \right\}^{1/2}},$$

where $\widehat{x_0} = f^{-1}(\overline{y_0}, \widehat{\theta})$ and $\widehat{S}^* = S_{\widehat{\theta}^*}$ is calculated at the x value $\widehat{x}^* = f^{-1}(\overline{y_0}^*, \widehat{\theta}^*)$. As a result, we obtain B values $\widehat{T}^{*,b}$, $b = 1, \ldots B$ of the bootstrap statistic. Let b_α be the α percentile of the $\widehat{T}^{*,b}$ (the method of calculating b_α was detailed in Section 2.4.1). This gives a bootstrap calibration interval for x_0 of

$$\widehat{J}_B = \left\{ x, \quad b_{\alpha/2} \widehat{S}_{\widehat{f}} \le \overline{y_0} - f(x, \widehat{\theta}) \le b_{1-\alpha/2} \widehat{S}_{\widehat{f}} \right\}, \tag{5.6}$$

where $\widehat{S}_{\widehat{f}}$ is defined in Equation (5.3). If, for example, f is strictly increasing, we can explicitly compute the bounds of the interval:

$$\widehat{J}_B = \left[f^{-1}\left(\overline{y_0} - b_{1-\alpha/2} \widehat{S}_{\widehat{f}}, \widehat{\theta} \right), \quad f^{-1}\left(\overline{y_0} - b_{\alpha/2} \widehat{S}_{\widehat{f}}, \widehat{\theta} \right) \right].$$

From the asymptotic theory, we know that the coverage probability of $\widehat{J}_B$ is close to $1 - \alpha$ for large n and B. In practice, with small sample sizes and B around 200, for example, $\widehat{J}_B$ has proved to behave reasonably well.

Likelihood Ratio Calibration Intervals

An alternative to bootstrap intervals is likelihood ratio intervals. These intervals are based on likelihood ratio test statistics (see Section 2.3.3).

Recall that $\widehat{\theta}$ is the least squares estimator of θ, that is, it minimizes the sum of squares

$$C(\theta) = \sum_{i=1}^{k} \sum_{j=1}^{n_i} (Y_{ij} - f(x_i, \theta))^2 \,.$$

The idea is to compare $C(\widehat{\theta})$ with the value of the sum of squares when θ is estimated subject to a known value of x_0. To define the confidence interval, assume that x_0 is known and compute the value of the parameter θ that minimizes the sum of squares defined by

$$\widetilde{C}(\theta) = \sum_{i=1}^{k} \sum_{j=1}^{n_i} (Y_{ij} - f(x_i, \theta))^2 + \sum_{l=1}^{m} (y_{0l} - f(x_0, \theta))^2 \,.$$

Let $\widetilde{\theta}$ denote this value. With these notations, the distribution of the statistic

$$\mathcal{S}_L = (n + m) \left\{ \log \widetilde{C}(\widetilde{\theta}) - \log \left(C(\widehat{\theta}) + \sum_{l=1}^{m} (y_{0l} - \overline{y_0})^2 \right) \right\}$$

can be approximated by a χ^2 with one degree of freedom. Equivalently, we can compute the signed root of $\mathcal{S}_L$ defined as

$$R_L(x_0) = \text{sign}\left(\overline{y_0} - f(x_0, \widehat{\theta}) \right) \sqrt{\mathcal{S}_L}.$$

The limiting distribution of R_L is an $\mathcal{N}(0, 1)$ distribution. We can deduce a confidence region for x_0 with asymptotic level $1 - \alpha$:

$$\widehat{J}_R = \left\{ x, \quad \nu_{\alpha/2} \le R_L(x) \le \nu_{1-\alpha/2} \right\}. \tag{5.7}$$

We use some numerical computations to obtain the endpoints of $\widehat{J}_R$.

Like $\widehat{J}_B$, $\widehat{J}_R$ has proved to perform well in practice. Its coverage probability is close to the desired confidence level.

5.3.3 Calibration with Nonconstant Variances

We saw in Chapter 3 that, in the case of heterogeneous variances, the appropriate estimation method is the maximum likelihood method. Recall that the log-likelihood based on observations Y_{ij} is

$$\log L_n \left(Y_{11}, \ldots, Y_{kn_k}, \theta, \sigma^2, \tau \right) =$$
$$-\frac{n}{2} \log 2\pi - \frac{1}{2} \sum_{i=1}^{k} \left[n_i \log \left(\sigma^2 g(x_i, \theta, \tau) \right) + \frac{\sum_{j=1}^{n_i} (Y_{ij} - f(x_i, \theta))^2}{\sigma^2 g(x_i, \theta, \tau)} \right].$$

Adding to the log-likelihood the observations y_{0l}, $l = 1, \ldots, m$, we obtain the global log-likelihood corresponding to our calibration model

$$V\left(\theta, \sigma^2, \tau, x_0\right) = \log L_n\left(Y_{11}, \ldots, Y_{kn_k}, \theta, \sigma^2, \tau\right)$$

$$-\frac{m}{2}\log 2\pi - \frac{m}{2}\log\left(\sigma^2 g(x_0, \theta, \tau)\right) - \frac{1}{2}\frac{\sum_{l=1}^{m}\left(y_{0l} - f(x_0, \theta)\right)^2}{\sigma^2 g(x_0, \theta, \tau)}.$$

Let $\widehat{\theta}, \widehat{\sigma}^2, \widehat{\tau}, \widehat{x_0}$ be the maximum likelihood estimators. A calibration interval for x_0 based on the asymptotic distribution of $\overline{y_0} - f(x_0, \widehat{\theta})$ is then just $\widehat{J}_\mathcal{N}$.

We can also, and this is what we recommend, compute a calibration interval based on the log-likelihood ratio (see Section 3.4.5). That is, we construct an analogous calibration interval as $\widehat{J}_R$ in the case of nonconstant variances. Compute $\widetilde{\theta}, \widetilde{\sigma}^2, \widetilde{\tau}$ that maximize $V(\theta, \sigma^2, \tau, x_0)$ given a fixed value of x_0. With these notations, the distribution of the statistic

$$R_L(x_0) = \text{sign}\left(\overline{y_0} - f(x_0, \widehat{\theta})\right) \times$$

$$\left\{2V\left(\widehat{\theta}, \widehat{\sigma}^2, \widehat{\tau}, \widehat{x_0}\right) - 2V\left(\widetilde{\theta}, \widetilde{\sigma}^2, \widetilde{\tau}, x_0\right)\right\}^{1/2}$$

can be approximated by an $\mathcal{N}(0,1)$ distribution. We can find a confidence interval for x_0 with asymptotic level $1 - \alpha$:

$$\widehat{J}_R = \left\{x, \quad \nu_{\alpha/2} \le R_L(x) \le \nu_{1-\alpha/2}\right\}. \tag{5.8}$$

Alternatively, we can propose bootstrap calibration intervals using the bootstrap resampling scheme presented in Section 3.4.3 combined with the method of computing a bootstrap calibration interval presented in Section 5.3.2.

5.4 Applications

5.4.1 Pasture Regrowth Example: Prediction of the Yield at Time $x_0 = 50$

Model The regression function used to analyze the pasture regrowth example (see Section 1.1.1) is

$$f(x, \theta) = \theta_1 - \theta_2 \exp\left(-\exp(\theta_3 + \theta_4 \log x)\right),$$

and the variances are homogeneous: $\text{Var}(\varepsilon_i) = \sigma^2$.

Results The adjusted response curve is

$$f(x, \widehat{\theta}) = 69.95 - 61.68 \exp\left(-\exp(-9.209 + 2.378 \log x)\right).$$

Calculation of Prediction Intervals for y_0 with Asymptotic Level 95% (See Equation (5.2))

$\widehat{y_0}$	$\left\{\widehat{\sigma}^2 + \widehat{S}^2\right\}^{1/2}$	$\nu_{0.975}$	$\widehat{I}_\mathcal{N}(x_0)$
49.37	1.17	1.96	[47.08 , 51.67]

Calculation of Prediction Intervals for y_0 with Asymptotic Level 95%, Using Bootstrap (See Equation (5.4))

The number of bootstrap simulations is $B=199$.

$\widehat{y}_0$	$\left\{\widehat{\sigma}^2 + \widehat{S}^2\right\}^{1/2}$	$b_{0.025}$	$b_{0.975}$	$\widehat{I}_B(x_0)$
49.37	1.17	-1.21	1.65	[47.96 , 51.31]

In this example, the two methods yield the same results: The prediction interval based on normal quantiles and the prediction interval based on bootstrap quantiles are nearly the same. The bootstrap quantiles catch some asymmetry of the distribution of $\widehat{T}$, but this has little effect on the result due to the small values of $\widehat{\sigma}$ and $\widehat{S}$. The numerical difference between the two intervals is due mainly to the variability between bootstrap simulations.

5.4.2 Cortisol Assay Example

Model In Chapter 4, we concluded that a satisfying model to analyze the cortisol assay data was based on an asymmetric sigmoidally shaped regression function

$$f(x,\theta) = \theta_1 + \frac{\theta_2 - \theta_1}{(1 + \exp(\theta_3 + \theta_4 x))^{\theta_5}}$$

with heteroscedastic variances $\mathrm{Var}(\varepsilon_{ij}) = \sigma^2 f^2(x_i, \theta)$.

Method The parameters are estimated by maximizing the log-likelihood; see Section 3.3.

Results The maximum likelihood estimators of the parameters are:

Parameters	Estimated Values
θ_1	133.42
θ_2	2758.7
θ_3	3.2011
θ_4	3.2619
θ_5	0.6084
σ^2	0.0008689

The calibration curve describes the relationship between the dose $d = 10^x$ and the expected response:

$$f\left(d, \widehat{\theta}\right) = \frac{2758.7 - 133.4}{(1 + \exp(3.2011 + 3.2619 \log_{10}(d)))^{0.6084}}.$$

The parameter of interest is the unknown dose of hormone d corresponding to the responses obtained from the following new experiment:

New Experiment	Response (c.p.m.)			
d?	2144	2187	2325	2330

Because we have nonconstant variances, we compute a likelihood ratio calibration interval and apply the results of Section 5.3.3 with $x_0 = d$.

Calculation of a Calibration Interval for d, with Asymptotic Level 95% (See Equation (5.8))

$\hat{d}$	$\hat{J}_R$
0.0574	[0.0516 , 0.0642]

$\hat{J}_R$ takes into account both the variability of the responses observed at dose d and the uncertainty about the calibration curve.

Bootstrap Calibration Interval We get the following result, based on $B = 500$ bootstrap simulations.

$\hat{d}$	$\hat{J}_R$
0.0574	[0.0524 , 0.0648]

5.4.3 Nasturtium Assay Example

Model The regression function is

$$f(x, \theta) = \theta_1 / (1 + \exp(\theta_2 + \theta_3 \log(x))),$$

and the variances are homogeneous: $\text{Var}(\varepsilon_i) = \sigma^2$.

Method The parameters are estimated by minimizing the sum of squares, $C(\theta)$; see Equation (1.10).

Results The calibration curve is defined by the following equation:

$$f\left(x, \widehat{\theta}\right) = \frac{897.86}{1 + \exp(-0.61 + 1.35 \log(x))}$$

and is shown in Figure 5.2.

Calculation of a Calibration Interval for the Unknown x_0 Corresponding to the Responses from the New Experiment (See Table 5.2) In the case of homogeneous variances, we proposed two calibration intervals. The first one, Equation (5.6), is based on bootstrap simulations; the second one, Equation (5.7), is based on the computation of the likelihood ratio statistic.

Bootstrap Interval In this example, 500 simulations of bootstrap samples ($B = 500$) are necessary to stabilize the values of the bootstrap percentiles. The following calibration interval was obtained from 500 bootstrap simulations:

$\widehat{x_0}$	$b_{0.025}$	$b_{0.975}$	$\hat{J}_B$
2.26	−1.55	1.50	[1.88 , 2.73]

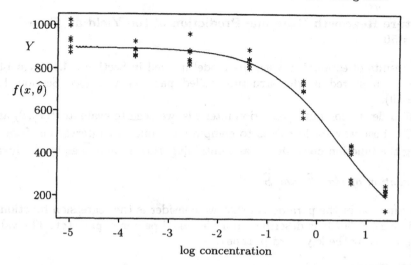

Figure 5.2. Nasturtium example: Graph of observed and adjusted response values

Likelihood Ratio Interval

$\widehat{x_0}$	$\widehat{J_R}$
2.26	[1.95 , 2.80]

The two methods do not yield the same result; but we have no argument to prefer one calibration interval over the other.

Note that in this example, the computation of the calibration interval $\widehat{J_N}$, according to Equation (5.5), yields [1.80, 2.91], which is wider than $\widehat{J_B}$ or $\widehat{J_R}$. This is not always the case. As already mentioned, $\widehat{J_B}$ or $\widehat{J_R}$ is to be preferred, both on theoretical grounds and from the results of simulation studies.

5.5 References

The theory underlying the construction of bootstrap and likelihood ratio calibration intervals can be found in [GHJ93] and [GJ94].

5.6 Using nls2

This section reproduces the commands and files used in this chapter to analyze the examples using **nls2**.

The commands introduced in earlier "Using **nls2**" sections are assumed to have already been executed.

Pasture Regrowth Example: Prediction of the Yield at Time $x_0 = 50$

The results of estimation with the model defined in Section 5.4.1, page 142, have been stored in the structure called **pasture.nl1** (see Section 1.6, page 19).

In order to compute prediction intervals, we need to evaluate $f(x_0, \widehat{\theta})$ and $\widehat{S}$. The best way to do this is to compute a confidence interval for $f(x_0, \theta)$ using the function **confidence** and obtaining $f(x_0, \widehat{\theta})$ and $\widehat{S}$ as by-products.

Calculation of $f(x_0, \widehat{\theta})$ and $\widehat{S}$

The function of the parameters that we consider is the regression function f at time $x_0 = 50$. It is described in a file called **pasture.predict**. The value of x_0 is set by the key word pbispsi:

```
psi yield;
ppsi p1, p2, p3, p4;
pbispsi x0;
subroutine;
begin
yield = p1-p2*exp(-exp(p3+p4*log(x0)));
end
```

We use the function **confidence** to compute the values of $f(x_0, \widehat{\theta})$ and $\widehat{S}$:

```
> pasture.conf.fx0<-confidence(pasture.nl1,
            file="pasture.predict",
            pbispsi=50)
>     # Print the results
> cat("Estimated value of f(x0,theta):", pasture.conf.fx0$psi,"\n" )
> cat("Estimated value of S:", pasture.conf.fx0$std.error,"\n" )
```

Prediction Interval $\widehat{I}_{\mathcal{N}}(x_0)$ for y_0, with Asymptotic Level 95%

From the previous results, we calculate the prediction interval $\widehat{I}_{\mathcal{N}}(x_0)$ for y_0 (see Equation (5.2), page 137):

```
> variance.y0 <- pasture.nl1$sigma2 + pasture.conf.fx0$var.psi
> sqrt.var <- sqrt(variance.y0)
> lower.y0<- pasture.conf.fx0$psi + qnorm(0.025)*sqrt.var
> upper.y0<- pasture.conf.fx0$psi + qnorm(0.975)*sqrt.var
```

We display the values of $\widehat{y_0}$, $\sqrt{\widehat{\sigma}^2 + \widehat{S}^2}$, $\nu_{0.975}$, and $\widehat{I}_{\mathcal{N}}(x_0)$:

```
> cat("Estimated value of y0:",pasture.conf.fx0$psi,"\n" )
> cat("Estimated value of the std:", sqrt.var,"\n" )
> cat("nu_(0.975):", qnorm(0.975),"\n" )
> cat("Estimated value of In:",lower.y0, upper.y0,"\n" )
```

Bootstrap Prediction Intervals for y_0

To calculate a bootstrap prediction interval for y_0, $\widehat{I}_B(x_0)$, according to Equation (5.4), page 139, we use the function **bootstrap** with the following option: **method="calib"**. This function returns the bootstrap percentiles of $\widehat{T}^*$:

```
> pasture.pred.y0<-bootstrap(pasture.nl1,
                            n.loops=500,
                            method="calib",
                            file="pasture.predict",
                            ord=pasture.conf.fx0$psi,
                            pbispsi=50)
> lower.y0<- pasture.conf.fx0$psi +
              pasture.pred.y0$conf.bounds[1] *sqrt(variance.y0)
> upper.y0<- pasture.conf.fx0$psi +
              pasture.pred.y0$conf.bounds[2] *sqrt(variance.y0)
```

We display the values of $\widehat{y}_0$, $b_{0.025}$, $b_{0.975}$, and $\widehat{I}_B(x_0)$:

```
> cat("Estimated value of y0:", pasture.conf.fx0$psi,"\n" )
> cat("b_0.025, b_0.975:",pasture.pred.y0$conf.bounds,"\n" )
> cat("Estimated value of Ib:",lower.y0,upper.y0,"\n" )
```

Note: The bootstrap method generates different numbers at each execution. Thus, results of these commands may vary slightly from those displayed in Section 5.4.1.

Cortisol Assay Example

The results of estimation when the regression function is an asymmetric sigmoidally shaped curve and the variances are heteroscedastic have been stored in the structure **corti.nl7** (see Section 4.6, page 125).

Likelihood Ratio Calibration Interval for x_0, with Asymptotic Level 95%

We use the function **calib** to calculate the calibration interval $\widehat{J}_R$ defined by Equation (5.8), page 142, for the unknown dose d of hormone that corresponds to the response values given in Section 5.4.2.

Before calling it, we have to:

1. Describe the inverse $f^{-1}(y, \theta)$ of the regression curve.
   We define it in a file called **corti.finv**:

```
abs dose;
ord f;
paract n,d,a,b,g;
pbisabs minf,pinf;
aux a1,a2,a3;
subroutine;
```

```
begin
a1 = (f-n)/(d-n);
a2 = exp(-(1/g)*log(a1));
a3 = (log(a2-1)-a)/b;
dose = if f >= d then minf else
       if f <= n then pinf else
       exp(a3*log(10))
fi   fi;
end
```

2. Generate the programs required by the function `calib`.
   The operating system commands `analDer`, `crCalib`, and `crInv` are provided with the system **nls2** to do that:
   - `analDer` generates the program that calculates the regression model.
   - `crCalib` generates the program that calculates d given fixed values of the regression parameters.
   - `crInv` generates the program that calculates the inverse of the regression curve.

   ```
   $ analDer corti.mod6
   $ crCalib corti.mod6
   $ crInv corti.finv
   ```

The programs required by the function `calib` are loaded into our S-Plus session by `loadnls2`. The environment variable `NLS2_DIR` is equal to the pathname of **nls2**. Then we apply `calib`. Using the option `x.bounds`, we specify a research interval:

```
> loadnls2(model=c("corti.mod6.c","corti.mod6.dc.c"),
         inv="corti.finv.c",
         tomyown=paste(getenv("NLS2_DIR"),"/EquNCalib.o", sep=""))
> corti.calib<-calib(corti.nl7,
         file="corti.finv",
         x.bounds=c(0.02,0.08),
         ord=c(2144,2187,2325,2330))
```

We display the values of $\widehat{d}$ and $\widehat{J}_R$:

```
> cat("Estimated value of d:", corti.calib$x,"\n" )
> cat("Jr:",corti.calib$R.conf.int,"\n" )
```

(Results are given in Section 5.4.2, page 143)

Nasturtium Assay Example

The nasturtium assay example is a new example, introduced in this chapter. We first create a *data frame* to store the experimental data. Then we estimate the parameters, and, finally, we calculate calibration intervals.

Creating the Data

The experimental data (see Table 5.1, page 136) are stored in a *data frame* called `nasturtium`:

```
> x.nas <-c(
 0.000,0.000,0.000,0.000,0.000,0.000,
 0.025,0.025,0.025,0.025,0.025,0.025,
 0.075,0.075,0.075,0.075,0.075,0.075,
 0.250,0.250,0.250,0.250,0.250,0.250,
 0.750,0.750,0.750,0.750,0.750,0.750,
 2.000,2.000,2.000,2.000,2.000,2.000,
 4.000,4.000,4.000,4.000,4.000,4.000)
> y.nas <-c(
 920,889,866,930,992,1017,919,878,882,854,851,850,870,825,953,
 834,810,875,880,834,795,837,834,810,693,690,722,738,563,591,
 429,395,435,412,273,257,200,244,209,225,128,221)
> nasturtium<-data.frame(x=x.nas,y=y.nas)
```

Plot of the Observed Weights Versus the Log Concentration

We plot the observed weights versus the log concentration. The zero concentration is represented by the value -5:

```
> log.nas<-c(rep(-5,6),log(x.nas[7:42]))
> plot(log.nas,y.nas,
        xlab="log-concentration",ylab="response",
        main="Nasturtium example",sub="Observed response")
```

(See Figure 5.1, page 136.)

Parameter Estimation

We describe the model defined by Equation (5.1), page 137, in a file called `nas.mod`:

```
resp y;
varind x;
parresp t1,t2,t3;
subroutine;
begin
y =  if x==0 then t1 else
     t1/(1+exp(t2+t3*log(x)))
          fi;
end
```

To estimate the parameters, we apply the function **nls2**. We plot the observed and fitted responses versus the log concentration using graphical functions of S-Plus. A line joins the fitted values:

```
> loadnls2() # reload the default programs
> nas.nl<-nls2(nasturtium,"nas.mod",c(900,-.5,1))
> plot(log.nas,y.nas,
        xlab="log-concentration",ylab="response",
        main="Nasturtium example",
        sub="Observed and adjusted response")
> lines(unique(log.nas),nas.nl$response)
```

(See Figure 5.2, page 145.)

Likelihood Ratio Calibration Interval for x_0 with Asymptotic Level 95%

To calculate the likelihood ratio calibration interval $\widehat{J}_R$ defined by Equation (5.7), page 141, for x_0, the unknown concentration that corresponds to the response values given in Table 5.2, page 136, we use the function `calib`.

In the cortisol example, additional programs were required to use `calib`. Here, the variances are homogeneous, and no extra work is necessary. We only have to describe the inverse of the regression function. We define it in a file called `nas.finv`:

```
abs x;
ord y;
paract t1,t2,t3;
aux a1;
subroutine;
begin
a1 = log( (t1/y) - 1) - t2;
x = if y >= t1 then 0 else
    exp( a1/t3 )
    fi;
end
```

We apply the function `calib` and display the values of $\log \widehat{x_0}$ and $\widehat{J}_R$:

```
> nas.calib<-calib(nas.nl, file = "nas.finv",
        ord=c(309, 296, 419))
>     # Print the results
> cat("Estimated value of x0:",  nas.calib$x,"\n" )
> cat("Jr:", nas.calib$R.conf.int,"\n" )
```

The calibration interval $\widehat{J}_N$ mentioned in the remark at the end of Section 5.4.3 is obtained as follows:

```
> cat("Jn:", nas.calib$S.conf.int,"\n" )
```

Bootstrap Calibration Interval for x_0

The function whose confidence interval is requested, i.e., the regression function f, is described in a file called `nas.psi`. The variable to be calibrated is introduced by the key word `pbispsi`:

```
psi y;
ppsi t1,t2,t3;
pbispsi x0;
subroutine;
begin
y =    t1/( 1 + exp( t2 + t3 * log(x0))  );
end
```

To calculate a confidence interval $\widehat{J}_B$ for x_0 according to Equation (5.6), page 140, we first use the function **bootstrap** with the argument **method** set to **calib**, which returns bootstrap percentiles, and then the function **calib**:

```
> nas.nl<-nls2(nasturtium,"nas.mod",c(900,-.5,1),renls2=T)
> nas.boot<-bootstrap(nas.nl,method="calib",file="nas.psi",
                      n.loops=500,
                      ord=c(309, 296, 419),
                      pbispsi=nas.calib$x)
> b0.025<-nas.boot$conf.bounds[1]
> b0.975<-nas.boot$conf.bounds[2]
> boot.calib<-calib(nas.nl,file="nas.finv",ord=c(309, 296, 419),
          conf.bounds=c(as.numeric(b0.025),as.numeric(b0.975)))
```

We display the values of $\widehat{x_0}$, $b_{0.025}$, $b_{0.975}$, and $\widehat{J}_B$:

```
> cat("Estimated value of x0:", boot.calib$x,"\n" )
> cat("b_0.025, b_0.975:",nas.boot$conf.bounds ,"\n" )
> cat("Estimated value of Jb:",boot.calib$S.conf.int,"\n" )
```

Results are displayed in Section 5.4.3, page 144. Note that bootstrap simulations generate different numbers at each execution, and the results of these commands may be slightly different from those reported in Section 5.4.3.

6

Binomial Nonlinear Models

This chapter extends the statistical methods used throughout the book to binomial response variables, with probability of response modeled as a nonlinear function of the independent variables.

Logistic regression models are special cases of binomial nonlinear models, where the probability of response is a monotone known function of a linear combination of the explanatory variables. Several of the examples given in this chapter fit into this framework, but they need a variety of extensions to the basic logistic model: The equation linking the probability of response to the independent variables is nonlinear in unknown parameters or the variance of the observations is not well modeled by the binomial variance (overdispersion). It is the aim of this chapter to present the extended models and show how to use **nls2** when dealing with them.

The text assumes a basic knowledge of estimation methods for generalized linear models based on maximum likelihood. Useful references are Collett [Col91], McCullagh and Nelder [MN89], Aitkin et al. [AAFH89], Chambers and Hastie [CH92], Venables and Ripley [VR94], and Dobson [Dob90].

6.1 Examples

6.1.1 Assay of an Insecticide with a Synergist: A Binomial Nonlinear Model

A typical experiment for assessing the tolerance of individuals to a toxic substance consists of applying different concentrations of the substance to several batches of individuals and recording the proportion of individuals giving an expected response. The data for this example have been treated by McCullagh and Nelder [MN89, page 384]. The aim of the experiment is the estimation of lowest-cost mixtures of insecticides and synergist. We observe the number Y_i of dead grasshoppers among N_i grasshoppers exposed to some doses of insecticide and synergist denoted, respectively, I_i and S_i. The results are reported in Table 6.1.

Table 6.1. Assay of an insecticide with a synergist

Dose of		Number	Total
Insecticide	Synergist	killed	number
4	0.0	7	100
5	0.0	59	200
8	0.0	115	300
10	0.0	149	300
15	0.0	178	300
20	0.0	229	300
2	3.9	5	100
5	3.9	43	100
10	3.9	76	100
2	19.5	4	100
5	19.5	57	100
10	19.5	83	100
2	39.0	6	100
5	39.0	57	100
10	39.0	84	100

The following model is assumed: The number of grasshoppers killed Y_i at doses $x_i = (I_i, S_i)$ is distributed as a binomial variable with parameters N_i and $p(x_i, \theta)$, where $p(x, \theta)$ describes the probability for an individual to die at doses x.

The model under study is the following:

$$Y_i \sim \mathcal{B}\left(N_i, p(x_i, \theta)\right).$$

In binomial linear models, it is assumed that the *probability function* $p(x, \theta)$ is related to a linear predictor η through a one-to-one transformation γ called the *link function*. Namely, $\gamma(p(x, \theta)) = \eta(x, \theta)$, where $\eta(x, \theta)$ is a linear function of θ. For example, take for all p in the interval $]0, 1[$

$$\gamma(p) = \text{logit}(p) = \log(p/(1-p))$$

and

$$\eta(x, \theta) = \theta_1 + \theta_2 I + \theta_3 S.$$

In our example, preliminary studies showed that the predictor η is not linear and led us to model the function η as follows:

$$\eta(x, \theta) = \text{logit}\left(p(x, \theta)\right) = \theta_1 + \theta_2 \log(I - \theta_3) + \theta_4 S/(\theta_5 + S). \quad (6.1)$$

Our aim is to estimate the parameters $\theta_1, \ldots, \theta_5$ and to evaluate the effect of doubling the dose of insecticide on the odds of a kill.

6.1.2 Vaso-Constriction in the Skin of the Digits: The Case of Binary Response Data

Let us continue with an example from Finney [Fin78] analyzed by Aitkin et al. [AAFH89]. The aim of the experiment is to study the effect of the rate and volume of air inspired on a transient vaso-constriction in the skin of the digits. The data are listed in Table 6.2. Three subjects were involved in the study. For each of them, the occurrence or nonoccurrence of vaso-constriction, as well as the rate and volume of air inspired, is measured several times: The response Y is set to 1 if vaso-constriction occurs and to 0 if not. For $i = 1, \ldots, k$ we denote by Y_i the response and by r_i and v_i the values of the variable rate and volume.

Table 6.2. Vaso-constriction in the skin of the digits

Volume	Rate	Response	Volume	Rate	Response
3.70	0.825	1	1.90	0.950	1
0.80	3.200	1	1.10	1.830	0
3.50	1.090	1	0.95	1.900	0
0.70	3.500	1	0.85	1.415	1
1.25	2.500	1	0.95	1.360	0
0.60	0.750	0	0.60	1.500	0
0.75	1.500	1	1.60	0.400	0
1.10	1.700	0	1.10	2.200	1
0.90	0.750	0	0.75	1.900	0
0.60	3.000	0	1.70	1.060	0
3.20	1.600	1	1.35	1.350	0
0.90	0.450	0	1.80	1.500	1
1.40	2.330	1	2.70	0.750	1
0.80	0.570	0	1.20	2.000	1
0.75	3.750	1	1.30	1.625	1
0.55	2.750	0	1.80	1.800	1
2.30	1.640	1	1.50	1.360	0
0.40	2.000	0	0.95	1.900	0
1.60	1.780	1	2.35	0.030	0
			0.80	3.330	1

In this example the variable rate and volume are not fixed in advance by the scientist but are the realization of random variables. Therefore we model the distribution of the response Y conditionally to the variables (r, v) as follows: Conditionally to the observed variable $x_i = (r_i, v_i)$, the response Y_i is distributed as a Bernoulli variable with parameter $p(x_i, \theta)$, where $p(x, \theta)$ denotes the probability for the vaso-constriction to occur conditionally to the fact that x is observed.

We will assume a logit-linear model, namely, $\text{logit}(p(x, \theta)) = \eta(x, \theta)$, where

$$\eta(x,\theta) = \theta_0 + \theta_1 \log(r) + \theta_2 \log(v).$$

This example has been extensively analyzed by Aitkin [AAFH89] and Pregibon [Pre81], especially for illustrating the use of diagnostic measures to detect lack of fit. We will only show how to estimate the parameters and compare two nested models using **nls2**.

6.1.3 Mortality of Confused Flour Beetles: The Choice of a Link Function in a Binomial Linear Model

Consider the following experiment that has already been extensively analyzed in the literature: See, for example, Collett [Col91, pages 109 and 140]. In this experiment, we observe the proportion of beetles killed versus the concentration of gaseous carbon disulphide (CS_2). Duplicate batches of beetles were used for each concentration. At the beginning of the experiment, for each i equals 1 to k and for each replicate $j = 1, 2$, N_{ij} beetles are exposed to a concentration of CS_2 equals to x_i. At the end of a five-hour period, the number of beetles killed Y_{ij} is recorded. The results are reported in Table 6.3 and Figure 6.1.

Table 6.3. Number of beetles killed, Y, out of beetles exposed, N, versus concentration of CS_2

Dose (mg/.1 ml)	First Replicate		Second Replicate	
	Y	N	Y	N
49.06	2	29	4	30
52.99	7	30	6	30
56.91	9	28	9	34
60.84	14	27	14	29
64.76	23	30	29	33
68.69	29	31	24	28
72.61	29	30	32	32
76.54	29	29	31	31

The following model is assumed: The number of killed beetles Y_{ij} at concentration x_i is distributed as a binomial variable with parameters N_{ij} and $p(x_i, \theta)$, where $p(x, \theta)$ describes the probability for an individual to die at concentration x.

The model under study is the following:

$$Y_{ij} \sim \mathcal{B}\left(N_{ij}, p(x_i, \theta)\right).$$

In this example, a possible choice for p is the Weibull function, presented in Section 1.1.1:

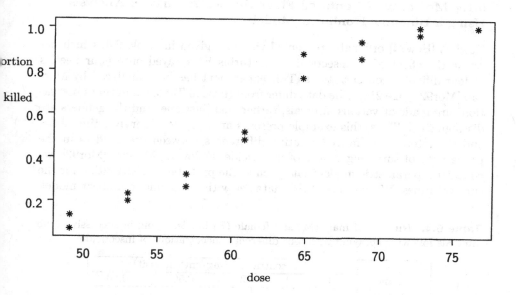

Figure 6.1. Beetles example: Observed frequencies versus the dose of CS2

$$p(x, \theta) = 1 - \exp(-\exp(\theta_1 + \theta_2 \log(x))).$$

This model is a binomial linear model, where the link function γ is defined as $\gamma(p) = \log(-\log(1 - p))$ and the linear predictor η equals $\eta(x, \theta) = \theta_1 + \theta_2 \log(x)$. The function γ is known as the complementary log-log function: $\gamma(p) = \text{cloglog}(p)$.

If the aim of this experiment is to estimate a dose that produces an extreme response, as, for example, the dose that produces death in 90% of the individuals exposed to it (termed the LD90), it is important to choose a model that fits the data well at extreme dose values. In this case, the choice of the link function γ may be of great importance. We will see how to choose γ using a family of parametric link functions. Namely, we will consider as link function the function:

$$\gamma(p, \theta_3) = \log\left(\frac{(1 - p)^{-\theta_3} - 1}{\theta_3}\right). \tag{6.2}$$

It is easy to verify that this family contains the logit link function (take $\theta_3 = 1$) and the cloglog link function (take $\theta_3 \to 0$). The parameter θ_3 being unknown, the model is a binomial nonlinear model, and we will see how to estimate simultaneously the parameters θ_1 to θ_3 and to calculate confidence intervals for the LD90.

6.1.4 Mortality of Confused Flour Beetles 2: Survival Analysis Using a Binomial Nonlinear Model

Hewlett [Hew74] originally presented the data given in Table 6.4, which describe the effect of an insecticide (Pyrethrins B) sprayed onto flour beetles at four different concentrations. This experiment has been analyzed by Morgan [Mor92, page 211]. The data differ from those in Table 6.3 in that observations are made at various intervals, rather than just one, and the genders are distinguished. Thus, this example presents an analysis of survival time data, and the interest lies in investigating differences between the genders in the probability of surviving a dose of insecticide. Following Morgan [Mor92], we consider a parametric model that specifies the probability distribution for the survival times. We will model this data set with a binomial nonlinear model.

Table 6.4. Number of male (M) and female (F) beetles dying in successive time intervals following spraying with four different concentrations of insecticide

Time interval (days)	Concentration (mg/cm^2 deposit)							
	0.20		0.32		0.50		0.80	
	M	F	M	F	M	F	M	F
0–1	3	0	7	1	5	0	4	2
1–2	11	2	10	5	8	4	10	7
2–3	10	4	11	11	11	6	8	15
3–4	7	8	16	10	15	6	14	9
4–5	4	9	3	5	4	3	8	3
5–6	3	3	2	1	2	1	2	4
6–7	2	0	1	0	1	1	1	1
7–8	1	0	0	1	1	4	0	1
8–9	0	0	0	0	0	0	0	0
9–10	0	0	0	0	0	0	1	1
10–11	0	0	0	0	0	0	0	0
11–12	1	0	0	0	0	1	0	0
12–13	1	0	0	0	0	1	0	0
No. treated	144	152	69	81	54	44	50	47

The observations are made of the number of male (M) and female (F) flour beetles Y_{ij} dying in the time interval (t_{j-1}, t_j) following spraying with a dose x_i, $i = 1, \ldots, 4$ of insecticide. N_i beetles are exposed at dose x_i. Let $p(x_i, t_j, \theta)$ describe the probability of a flour beetle dying at concentration x_i in the time interval (t_{j-1}, t_j). We assume that Y_{ij} is distributed as a binomial variable $\mathcal{B}(N_i, p(x_i, t_j, \theta))$. A possible choice for p proposed by Morgan [Mor92] is

$$p(x_i, t_j, \theta) = H(x_i, t_j, \theta) - H(x_i, t_j - 1, \theta),$$

where

$$H(x_i, t_j, \theta) = \frac{1}{1 + \exp(-\theta_1 - \theta_2 \log(x_i))} \times \frac{1}{1 + \exp(\theta_3 - \theta_4 \log(t_j))}.$$

The interpretation of the model is as follows: At dose level x_i a proportion $(1 + \exp(-\theta_1 - \theta_2 \log(x_i)))^{-1}$ of beetles are killed. These susceptible beetles will respond at various times, and the cumulative survival-time distribution $F(t) = \{1 + \exp(\theta_3 - \theta_4 \log(t))\}^{-1}$ for $t \geq 0$ and $\theta_4 > 0$ is independent of the dose.

We will see how to estimate the parameters and compare the distribution of time to death between the genders. We will show how the computations of this nonlinear survival analysis can be performed easily using **nls2**.

6.1.5 Germination of Orobranche: Overdispersion

We consider a data set originally presented by Crowder [Cro78]. The aim of the experiment is to evaluate the factors affecting the germination of the seed of two varieties of Orobranche cultivated in a dilution of two different extracts, a bean root extract and a cucumber root extract. The data are given in Table 6.5.

Table 6.5. Number of germinated seed, Y, out of N seeds

Species	O. aegyptiaca 75				O. aegyptiaca 73			
Extracts	Bean		Cucumber		Bean		Cucumber	
Y	N	Y	N	Y	N	Y	N
10	39	5	6	8	16	3	12
23	62	53	74	10	30	22	41
26	51	32	51	23	45	32	51
17	39	46	79	0	4	3	7
		10	13				

For i varying from 1 to 4 and for each replication j varying from 1 to n_i, we observe for the species S_i, the number of seeds germinated, Y_{ij}, among N_{ij} seeds brushed onto a plate containing a 1/125 dilution of an extract denoted by E_i. The variables (S, E) are qualitative variables defined as follows: $S = 0$ when the species is Orobranche aegyptiaca 75 and $S = 1$ when the species is Orobranche aegyptiaca 73, $E = 0$ if the Orobranche is cultivated on the bean root extract and $E = 1$ if it is cultivated on the cucumber root extract. In a first approach, the observation Y_{ij} is assumed to be distributed as a binomial variable $\mathcal{B}(N_{ij}, p(x_i, \theta))$, where $x_i = (S_i, E_i)$. Some preliminary analyses indicated that the main effects of species and extract as well as the interaction term should be retained in the model (Collett [Col91, page 191]). Therefore, the probability function corresponds to the saturated model in a 2×2 factorial experiment and is written as

$$\text{logit}\,(p(x_i, \theta)) = \theta_0 + \theta_1 S_i + \theta_2 E_i + \theta_3 S_i E_i.$$

We will see that these data are overdispersed. This means that the variance of the observation Y_{ij} is greater than can be expected on the basis of binomial sampling errors where

$$\text{Var}(Y_{ij}) = N_{ij} p(x_i, \theta)(1 - p(x_i, \theta)).$$

We will show how to treat the problem of overdispersion using the quasi-likelihood method available in **nls2**.

6.2 The Parametric Binomial Nonlinear Model

Let us introduce the following notation for defining the parametric binomial nonlinear model.

First, we consider the case of binary response that is either a failure or a success. Namely, we set $Y = 1$ when the response occurs and $Y = 0$ if not. In Example 6.1.2, Y is the occurrence of the vaso-constriction in the skin of the digit. In binary response data, for each value of the variable x_i, i varying from 1 to k, the response Y_i is observed. The variables $Y_i, i = 1, \ldots, k$, are assumed to be independent and distributed as a Bernoulli variable, such that $\Pr(Y_i = 1) = p(x_i, \theta)$.

Second, we consider the case of binomial response data. For each value of the variable x_i and for each replicate $j = 1, \ldots, n_i$, the responses of N_{ij} individuals are considered: For each l varying from 1 to N_{ij}, we denote by R_{ijl} the response of individual j. The R_{ijl}s are binary variables equal to 1 when the response occurs and 0 if not. The observation $Y_{ij} = \sum_{l=1}^{N_{ij}} R_{ijl}$ is the number of individuals out of N_{ij} for which the response occurs. In Example 6.1.1, i varies from 1 to $k = 15$, the numbers of replicate n_i are equal to 1, and N_i grasshoppers are exposed to some doses of insecticide and synergist x_i. The variable R_{il} equals 1 when a grasshopper dies, and Y_i is the number of dead grasshoppers among N_i.

If for $l = 1, \ldots, N_{ij}$, the responses R_{ijl} are independent Bernoulli variables with parameter $p(x_i, \theta)$, then the variable Y_{ij} is distributed as a binomial variable with parameters N_i and $p(x_i, \theta)$:

$$Y_{ij} \sim \mathcal{B}(N_{ij}, p(x_i, \theta)). \tag{6.3}$$

The probability function $p(x, \theta)$ depends on p unknown parameters θ. If $p(x, \theta)$ is related to a linear predictor η through a known link function γ, namely,

$$\gamma(p(x, \theta)) = \eta(x, \theta),$$

where η is a linear function of θ, then the model is a binomial linear model. This is the case in Examples 6.1.2 and 6.1.3 if the parameter θ_3 in Equation (6.2) is fixed to a known value. If such a relation does not exist, then the model is a binomial nonlinear model: In Example 6.1.1 the logit transform of $p(x, \theta)$ is a nonlinear function of the parameters; in Example 6.1.3 the function γ is known up to an unknown parameter θ_3; and in Example 6.1.4 the probability $p(x, \theta)$ is directly modeled as a nonlinear function of the parameters.

6.3 Overdispersion, Underdispersion

Let us recall that a binomial variable with parameters N and $p(x, \theta)$ is by definition the sum of N independent Bernoulli variables with parameter $p(x, \theta)$. It follows that there are many reasons for model misspecifications. This problem is discussed in detail by several authors (see, for example, Collett [Col91] and McCullagh and Nelder [MN89]) and is beyond the scope of this book. We will confine ourselves to making the link between the binomial nonlinear model and the heteroscedastic nonlinear regression model given by equations (3.7). Indeed, if we use a binomial nonlinear model to model the data set, then we get the following:

$$E(Y_{ij}) = N_{ij}p(x_i, \theta),$$
$$\text{Var}(Y_{ij}) = N_{ij}p(x_i, \theta)\left(1 - p(x_i, \theta)\right).$$

In some cases, it appears that the modeling of the variance function is not correct, although it is not clear how to improve the modeling of the probability function. We are thus led to propose other variance functions. Several models are proposed and briefly described here. They are illustrated with the Orobranche Example 6.1.5 (see Collett [Col91, Chapter 6] for more details).

Modeling the Variability in the Probability Function

If the different batches of seed were not germinated in the same experimental conditions, then the variance of the observation would increase by a constant factor denoted σ^2,

$$\text{Var}(Y_{ij}) = \sigma^2 N_{ij}p(x_i, \theta)\left(1 - p(x_i, \theta)\right). \tag{6.4}$$

More generally, if one relevant explanatory variable is not taken into account in the modeling of the probability function then the variation of the responses increases. To introduce variability in the probability function we consider a set of independent variables $(P_1, \ldots, P_k)$, with $E(P_i) = p(x_i, \theta)$ and $\text{Var}(P_i) = \tau p(x_i, \theta)\left(1 - p(x_i, \theta)\right)$, and we assume that conditional on $P_i = p(x_i, \theta)$, Y_{ij} is distributed as a binomial variable $\mathcal{B}\left(N_{ij}, p(x_i, \theta)\right)$.

Adding a random effect to the probability function leads us to consider a mixed effect model, where the distribution of Y_{ij} is a mixture of two distributions: The law of Y_{ij} is obtained by integrating the binomial distribution with respect to the law of the variable P_i. In fact we do not need to know the law of Y_{ij} because we will not estimate the parameters by maximizing the likelihood. We will use the quasi-likelihood method that requires knowledge of the moments of Y_{ij} only.

Some simple calculations lead to the following results:

$$\left.\begin{array}{l} \mathrm{E}(Y_{ij}) = N_{ij}p(x_i, \theta), \\ \mathrm{Var}(Y_{ij}) = N_{ij}p(x_i, \theta)\left(1 - p(x_i, \theta)\right)\left[1 + \tau(N_{ij} - 1)\right] \end{array}\right\}. \tag{6.5}$$

Several other models have been proposed; see Williams [Wil82]. For example, P_i is assumed to have a beta-distribution (Williams [Wil75], Crowder [Cro78]) leading to:

$$\left.\begin{array}{l} \mathrm{E}(Y_{ij}) = N_{ij}p(x_i, \theta), \\ \mathrm{Var}(Y_{ij}) = N_{ij}p(x_i, \theta)\left(1 - p(x_i, \theta)\right)\left[1 + \tau_i(N_{ij} - 1)\right] \end{array}\right\}, \tag{6.6}$$

where $\tau_1, \ldots, \tau_k$ are unknown parameters to estimate, or $\mathrm{logit}(P_i)$ is assumed to have a Gaussian distribution with expectation $\eta(x_i, \theta)$ and variance τ^2 leading to:

$$\left.\begin{array}{l} \mathrm{E}(Y_{ij}) \approx N_{ij}p(x_i, \theta), \\ \mathrm{Var}(Y_{ij}) \approx N_{ij}p(x_i, \theta)\left(1 - p(x_i, \theta)\right)\left[1 + \tau(N_{ij} - 1)p(x_i, \theta)\left(1 - p(x_i, \theta)\right)\right] \end{array}\right\}, \tag{6.7}$$

these last approximations are valid when the variance τ^2 is small. The variance functions defined by Equations (6.5) to (6.7) are not relevant when we observe binary data where all the N_{ij}s equal 1. In the same way, the variance function defined by Equation (6.6) is relevant only if for each $i = 1, \ldots, k$, some of the N_{ij}s are greater than 2. Indeed, if $N_{ij} = 1$ for all j, the parameter τ_i disappears and cannot be estimated.

Modeling Correlation in the Binary Individual Responses

If the germination of one seed in one particular batch promotes germination of the other seeds in the same batch, then the individual binary responses, $R_{ijl}, l = 1, \ldots, N_{ij}$, are correlated. Therefore the variable $Y_{ij} = \sum_{l=1}^{N_{ij}} R_{ijl}$ is no longer distributed as a binomial variable, and it can be shown that its variance may increase or decrease. Namely, if τ is the correlation coefficient between R_{ijl} and R_{ijk}, then the expectation and the variance of Y_{ij} are the same as those given by Equation (6.5) (see Collett [Col91, page 195]).

6.4 Estimation

6.4.1 Case of Binomial Nonlinear Models

If we consider the binomial nonlinear model described in Section 6.2, it is natural to estimate the parameters θ by maximizing the likelihood, because the distribution of the observations is known. We begin this section by introducing the deviance function because, in binomial linear models, it is more common to work with the deviance function than with the likelihood.

For i varying from 1 to k, the observed variables Y_{ij} are independent binomial variables with parameters N_{ij} and $p(x_i, \theta)$. The case of binary response data corresponds to $n_i = 1$ and $N_{ij} = 1$ for all $i = 1, \ldots k$.

The *deviance* is defined as:

$$D(\theta) = -2 \sum_{i=1}^{k} \sum_{j=1}^{n_i} Y_{ij} \log \left(\frac{N_{ij} p(x_i, \theta)}{Y_{ij}} \right) + (N_{ij} - Y_{ij}) \log \left(\frac{N_{ij} - N_{ij} p(x_i, \theta)}{N_{ij} - Y_{ij}} \right).$$

$$(6.8)$$

For a given set of observations $(Y_{ij}, j = 1, \ldots, n_i, i = 1, \ldots, k)$, the deviance is a function of the parameters. It can be shown that the *minimum deviance estimator* $\widehat{\theta}$ is the maximum likelihood estimator and that it is defined as a quasi-likelihood estimator (see Section 3.3.2). Namely, $\widehat{\theta}$ satisfies $U_a(\widehat{\theta}) = 0$, for $a = 1, \ldots, p$, where

$$U_a(\theta) = \sum_{i=1}^{k} \sum_{j=1}^{n_i} \frac{Y_{ij} - N_{ij} p(x_i, \theta)}{p(x_i, \theta)\,(1 - p(x_i, \theta))} \frac{\partial p}{\partial \theta_a}(x_i, \theta). \qquad (6.9)$$

For calculating the maximum likelihood estimator of θ using **nls2**, we will use the quasi-likelihood method (see Section 6.7).

Let us briefly recall how the deviance is calculated in a binomial model. For Y a random variable distributed as a $\mathcal{B}(N, p)$, we set

$$\ell(y, N, p) = \Pr(Y = y) = \frac{N!}{y!(N-y)!} p^y (1-p)^{N-y}.$$

Let us denote by $\tilde{Y}$ the vector of observations:

$$\tilde{Y} = (Y_{11}, \ldots, Y_{1n_1}, \ldots, Y_{k1}, \ldots, Y_{kn_k})^T,$$

and by $\tilde{p}$ the vector of probabilities. The components of $\tilde{p}$ are denoted p_{ij}, for $i = 1, \ldots, k$ and $j = 1, \ldots, n_i$. Each p_{ij} is the expectation of Y_{ij}/N_{ij}. When the probability function is such that $p_{ij} = p(x_i, \theta)$ for all $j = 1, \ldots, n_i$, then the quantities $p(x_i, \theta)$ are replicated n_i times in order to compose a vector denoted by $\tilde{p}(\theta)$ with $n = \sum_{i=1}^{k} n_i$ components.

The likelihood function is defined by the following formula:

$$L\left(\tilde{Y}, \tilde{p}\right) = \prod_{i=1}^{k} \prod_{j=1}^{n_i} \ell(Y_{ij}, N_{ij}, p_{ij}).$$

For i varying from 1 to k and for j from 1 to n_i, let

$$\pi_{ij} = \frac{Y_{ij}}{N_{ij}}$$

be the empirical frequencies. Note that in a binary response model, $\pi_i = Y_i$. Then, for a given model of the probability function, $p_{ij} = p(x_i, \theta)$, the deviance is defined as follows:

$$D(\theta) = -2 \log \frac{L\left(\tilde{Y}, \tilde{p}(\theta)\right)}{L\left(\tilde{Y}, \tilde{\pi}\right)}.$$

It is easy to verify that it is exactly what Equation (6.8) states. Moreover, it is clear that minimizing $D(\theta)$ is equivalent to maximizing $L\left(\tilde{Y}, \tilde{p}(\theta)\right)$.

The link between minimum of deviance estimation and quasi-likelihood estimation is done by noting that minimizing $D(\theta)$ is equivalent to solving the estimating equations defined by the following:

$$\frac{\partial D}{\partial \theta_a}(\theta) = 0, \text{ for } a = 1, \dots, p.$$

Starting from Equation (6.8), we get

$$\frac{\partial D}{\partial \theta_a}(\theta) = -2 \sum_{i=1}^{k} \sum_{j=1}^{n_i} \frac{Y_{ij}}{p(x_i, \theta)} \frac{\partial p}{\partial \theta_a}(x_i, \theta) - \frac{N_{ij} - Y_{ij}}{1 - p(x_i, \theta)} \frac{\partial p}{\partial \theta_a}(x_i, \theta).$$

It is easy to verify that

$$\frac{\partial D}{\partial \theta_a}(\theta) = -2U_a(\theta),$$

where $U_a(\theta)$ is defined by Equation (6.9).

6.4.2 Case of Overdispersion or Underdispersion

We consider the nonlinear model defined by

$$\left.\begin{array}{l} \mathrm{E}(Y_{ij}) = N_{ij} p(x_i, \theta), \\ \mathrm{Var}(Y_{ij}) = \sigma^2 g(x_i, N_{ij}; \theta, \tau) \end{array}\right\}, \tag{6.10}$$

where g is the variance function. If the Y_{ij}s are binomial variables, then $\sigma^2 = 1$, g depends on θ only, and

$$g(x, N; \theta, \tau) = g(x, N; \theta) = Np(x, \theta)(1 - p(x, \theta)).$$

Overdispersion or underdispersion for the binomial case may be treated by estimating σ^2 and the additional parameter τ. In case (6.4), σ^2 is estimated by the residual variance:

$$\widehat{\sigma}^2 = \frac{1}{n} \sum_{i=1}^{k} \sum_{j=1}^{n_i} \frac{\left(Y_{ij} - N_{ij} p(x_i, \widehat{\theta})\right)^2}{N_{ij} p(x_i, \widehat{\theta}) \left(1 - p(x_i, \widehat{\theta})\right)}. \tag{6.11}$$

In cases (6.5) to (6.7), $\sigma^2 = 1$ and q parameters τ have to be estimated, where $q = 1$ in cases (6.5) and (6.7) and $q = k$ in case (6.6). For this purpose, we use the quasi-likelihood method defined in Section 3.3.2. The quasi-likelihood equations are given by the following formulas:

$$U_a(\theta, \tau) = \sum_{i=1}^{k} \sum_{j=1}^{n_i} \frac{Y_{ij} - N_{ij} p(x_i, \theta)}{g(x_i, N_{ij}; \theta, \tau)} N_{ij} \frac{\partial p}{\partial \theta_a}(x_i, \theta), \text{ for } a = 1, \dots, p,$$

$$U_{p+b}(\theta, \tau) = \sum_{i=1}^{k} \sum_{j=1}^{n_i} \frac{(Y_{ij} - N_{ij} p(x_i, \theta))^2 - \sigma^2 g(x_i, N_{ij}; \theta, \tau)}{g^2(x_i, N_{ij}; \theta, \tau)} \frac{\partial g}{\partial \tau_b}(x_i, N_{ij}; \theta, \tau)$$

for $b = 1, \ldots, q$.

The choice of the weights introduced in the quasi-likelihood equations can be explained as follows: For $a = 1, \ldots, p$, the weight function $g(x_i, N_{ij}; \theta, \tau)$ in $U_a(\theta, \tau)$ is proportional to the variance of $Y_{ij} - N_{ij} p(x_i, \theta)$ (see Equation (6.10)); for $b = 1, \ldots, q$, the choice of the weights in U_{p+b} is justified by an asymptotic argument. It is known by the central limit theorem that if Z is the sum of N identically distributed variables with expectation μ and variance σ^2, then, when N is large, the distribution of $(Z - N\mu)/\sqrt{N}\dot{\sigma}$ can be approximated by the centered Gaussian distribution with variance 1. Therefore the quasi-likelihood equations are constructed as if the moments up to the order 4, of the variables ε_{ij} defined as

$$E(\varepsilon_{ij}^\ell) = E\left((Y_{ij} - N_{ij} p(x_i, \theta))^\ell \right),$$

for $\ell = 1, \ldots, 4$, were equal to the moments of centered Gaussian variables with variance equal to $\sigma^2 g(X_i, N_{ij}; \theta, \tau)$. It follows that if N_{ij} is large enough,

$$\mathrm{Var}\left((Y_{ij} - N_{ij} p(x_i, \theta))^2 \right) \approx 2\sigma^4 g^2(X_i, N_{ij}; \theta, \tau).$$

6.5 Tests and Confidence Regions

The methods for testing hypotheses or calculating confidence intervals for models defined in Section 6.2 are similar to those described in Section 3.4 for heteroscedastic nonlinear models. For any continuous function of the parameters $\lambda(\theta, \sigma^2, \tau)$ we can test hypothesis H: $\lambda = \lambda_0$ against the alternative A: $\lambda \neq \lambda_0$ using the Wald statistic S_W as described in Section 3.4.1.

The bootstrap estimation of λ is based on estimates $\widehat{\lambda}^*$ calculated exactly as in Section 3.4.3.

The likelihood ratio tests for comparing nested models or calculating confidence regions can be applied as in Sections 3.4.2 and 3.4.5. Nevertheless, in binomial models the test statistic is usually calculated using the deviance function. Therefore we will present the tests based on the deviance function in this chapter.

Likelihood Ratio Tests and Confidence Regions Using the Deviance Function

In Section 3.4.2, the likelihood ratio test statistic was introduced for the Gaussian regression model. The same process applies to the binomial nonlinear regression model using the deviance statistic in place of the likelihood ratio statistic. We consider the model described in Equation (6.3), for some probability function $p(x, \theta)$ that depends on p unknown parameters θ.

We consider the situation where a hypothesis H is described by a linear constraint on a subset of the parameter vector θ. The constraint is expressed as $\Lambda\theta = L_0$, where Λ is an $r \times p$ matrix $(r \leq p)$ of rank r, and L_0 is a constant vector with dimension r. Let $\widehat{\theta}_{\mathrm{H}}$ be the maximum likelihood estimator of θ under hypothesis H, and let $\widehat{\theta}$ be the maximum likelihood estimator under the alternative that there is no constraint on the parameters. The likelihood ratio test statistic is

$$\mathcal{S}_{\mathrm{L}} = D(\widehat{\theta}_{\mathrm{H}}) - D(\widehat{\theta}).$$

Following Equation (6.8), this turns out to be:

$$\mathcal{S}_{\mathrm{L}} = -2 \sum_{i=1}^{k} \sum_{j=1}^{n_i} Y_{ij} \log\left(\frac{p(x_i, \widehat{\theta}_{\mathrm{H}})}{p(x_i, \widehat{\theta})}\right) + (N_{ij} - Y_{ij}) \log\left(\frac{1 - p(x_i, \widehat{\theta}_{\mathrm{H}})}{1 - p(x_i, \widehat{\theta})}\right).$$

Hypothesis H is rejected if $\mathcal{S}_{\mathrm{L}} > C$, where C is defined by

$$\Pr\{Z_r \le C\} = 1 - \alpha.$$

Z_r is distributed as a χ^2 with r degrees of freedom, and α is the (asymptotic) level of the test.

Let us specify what *asymptotic* means. If we observe binary data, then *asymptotic* means that the number of observations k tends to infinity. If we observe binomial data, then the meaning of *asymptotic* depends on the modeling of the probability function p.

Consider Example 6.1.1, where for each dose x_i, $i = 1, \ldots, k$, we observe Y_i, the number of dead grasshoppers among N_i. The probability function described in Equation (6.1) depends on p parameters. This number p is fixed ($p = 5$) and does not increase with k. Therefore we can consider two cases: *Asymptotic* means that the number of observations k tends to infinity, or *asymptotic* means that for each $i = 1, \ldots, k$, N_i tends to infinity.

In Example 6.1.5, for i varying from 1 to k ($k = 4$) we observe for the modality (S_i, E_i) of the explanatory variables, n_i replications of the number of seeds germinated Y_{ij}, among N_{ij}. The probability function corresponds to the saturated model in a 2×2 factorial experiment and the number of parameters to estimate equals k: estimating the parameters $\theta_0, \ldots, \theta_3$ is equivalent to estimating the probabilities $p((0, 0), \theta)$, $p((0, 1), \theta)$, $p((1, 0), \theta)$, and $p((1, 1), \theta)$. In that case *asymptotic* means that for each $i = 1, \ldots, k$, $\sum_{i=1}^{n_i} N_{ij}$ tends to infinity. Note that in the case of no replication, when $n_i = 1$, then *asymptotic* means that N_i tends to infinity.

In the same way we calculated confidence regions based on the maximum likelihood approach in Section 3.4.5, we can compute *confidence intervals* or *confidence regions using the deviance*. Let us denote by $\mathcal{S}_{\mathrm{L}}(L_0)$ the test statistic of hypothesis H against alternative A, then the set of vectors L_0 with r components such that $\mathcal{S}_{\mathrm{L}}(L_0) > C$ is a confidence region for $\Lambda\theta$ with (asymptotic) level α.

The comparison of two nested models is done as in Section 4.3.1. Consider hypothesis A, where the probability function $p(x, \theta)$ depends on p_{A} parameters, and hypothesis H such that the model associated with H is nested into the model associated with A and where the probability function $p(x, \theta)$ depends on p_{H} parameters, $p_{\mathrm{H}} < p_{\mathrm{A}}$. In Example 6.1.3, for testing that the link function is the logit function, we compare the model associated with hypothesis A and defined by Equation (6.2) to the model associated with hypothesis

H defined by the constraint $\theta_3 = 1$. Let $\widehat{\theta}_H$ and $\widehat{\theta}_A$ be the maximum likelihood estimators under hypotheses H and A, respectively, then the test statistic equals:

$$S_L = D(\widehat{\theta}_H) - D(\widehat{\theta}_A),$$ (6.12)

and hypothesis H is rejected if $S_L > C$, where C satisfies

$$\Pr\{Z_{p_A - p_H} \leq C\} = 1 - \alpha.$$

Goodness-of-Fit Test

Let us consider the binomial nonlinear model described in Equation (6.3) where the dimension of the parameter θ equals p, and where the maximum likelihood estimator of the parameters is denoted by $\widehat{\theta}$. Assume that for each $i = 1, \ldots, k$, and $j = 1, \ldots, n_i$, the quantities N_{ij} are large.

Testing goodness of fit consists of testing the model (6.3) against the saturated model defined by

$$Y_{ij} \sim \mathcal{B}(N_{ij}, p_{ij}),$$ (6.13)

where the p_{ij}s are the $n = \sum_{i=1}^{k} n_i$ parameters of the model. The maximum likelihood estimators of the probabilities p_{ij} are the empirical frequencies $\pi_{ij} = Y_{ij}/N_{ij}$, and the likelihood ratio test statistic is simply the deviance associated with model (6.3). Therefore the hypothesis that the model is defined by (6.3) against the alternative that it is defined by (6.13) is rejected when the deviance $D(\widehat{\theta})$ is greater than C where C satisfies

$$\Pr\{Z_{n-p} \leq C\} = 1 - \alpha.$$

The properties of the goodness-of-fit test are known when for each $i = 1, \ldots, k$ and $j = 1, \ldots, n_i$, N_{ij} tends to infinity. Then, the asymptotic level of the test is equal to α and the power of the test tends to 1. Note that in the case of binary data, it is not possible to test goodness of fit.

6.6 Applications

6.6.1 Assay of an Insecticide with a Synergist: Estimating the Parameters

Model The observations are binomial variables, $Y_i \sim \mathcal{B}(N_i, p(x_i, \theta))$, and the probability function is

$$\text{logit}(p(x_i, \theta)) = \theta_1 + \theta_2 \log(I_i - \theta_3) + \theta_4 S_i/(\theta_5 + S_i).$$ (6.14)

The definition of the model is complete if the parameters θ satisfy the following constraints: $I - \theta_3$ and θ_5 must be strictly positive.

Method The parameters are estimated by minimizing the deviance $D(\theta)$; see Equation (6.8).

Results

Parameters	Estimated Values	Standard Error
θ_1	-2.89	0.24
θ_2	1.34	0.10
θ_3	1.67	0.11
θ_4	1.71	0.17
θ_5	2.06	1.09

Goodness-of-Fit Test and Graphics for Diagnostic The minimum deviance $D(\widehat{\theta})$ equals 18.7. Using the results of Section 6.5, we test the hypothesis that the probability function is the function defined by Equation (6.14) with $p = 5$ parameters against the alternative that $p(x_i, \theta) = \pi_i$ with $k = 15$ parameters. The condition that the N_is are large is satisfied, because all the N_is are greater than 100. The 95% quantile of a χ^2 variable with $k - p = 10$ degrees of freedom being equal to 18.3, the goodness-of-fit test based on the deviance with an asymptotic 5% level is rejected. This result would lead us to reject model (6.14). Nevertheless, the value of the statistic is very close to the critical value, and it is more appropriate to conclude by noting that the probability for a χ^2 variable with ten degrees of freedom to be greater than 18.7 equals 4.5%.

As explained in Chapter 4, model misspecifications can be detected by examining the data together with the results of the estimation (see Collett [Col91, Chapter 5] for a complete description of model checking for binomial data). The plot of fitted $p(x, \widehat{\theta})$ versus x_i or observed frequencies, and the plots of residuals are useful tools for assessing the quality of the fit. The *deviance residuals* and the *Pearson residuals* are usually calculated. They are defined as follows: For each i and j, let

$$\widehat{d}_{ij} = -2\left[Y_{ij}\log\left(N_{ij}p(x_i,\widehat{\theta})\right) + (N_{ij} - Y_{ij})\log\left(\frac{N_{ij} - N_{ij}p(x_i,\widehat{\theta})}{N_{ij} - Y_{ij}}\right)\right],$$

then the deviance residuals $\widehat{r}_{ij}$ are defined by:

$$\widehat{r}_{ij} = \text{sign}(Y_{ij} - N_{ij}p(x_i,\widehat{\theta}))\sqrt{\widehat{d}_{ij}}. \tag{6.15}$$

It is easy to verify that $D(\widehat{\theta}) = \sum_{i=1}^{k}\sum_{j=1}^{n_i}(\widehat{r}_{ij})^2$. The Pearson residuals are the standardized residuals defined as follows:

$$\widehat{e}_{ij} = \frac{Y_{ij} - N_{ij}p(x_i,\widehat{\theta})}{\sqrt{N_{ij}p(x_i,\widehat{\theta})\left(1 - p(x_i,\widehat{\theta})\right)}}.$$

The adjusted probability function, $p(x, \widehat{\theta})$, versus the observed frequencies is shown in Figure 6.2. The plots of deviance and Pearson residuals are shown in Figure 6.3. In this example the deviance and Pearson residuals are similar. Two points have residuals greater than two in absolute value. They correspond to a null dose of synergist and small doses of insecticide 4 and 5. These figures do not show any particular model misspecification.

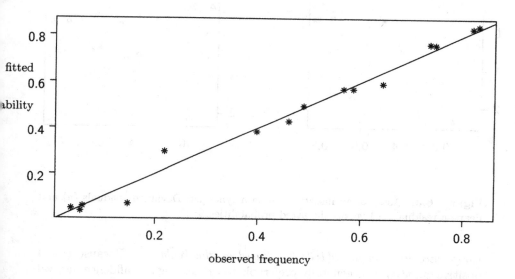

Figure 6.2. Assay of an insecticide with a synergist: Graph of adjusted probabilities versus observed frequencies

Confidence Interval for the Odds Ratio When the Dose of Insecticide is Doubled The odds of an insect dying when it is exposed to a dose $x = (I, S)$ of insecticide and synergist is

$$o(I, S) = p(x, \theta)/(1 - p(x, \theta))$$
$$= \exp\{\theta_1 + \theta_2 \log(I - \theta_3) + \theta_4 S/(\theta_5 + S)\}.$$

The odds ratio when doubling the dose of insecticide is the ratio of the odds of an insect exposed to a dose $(2I, S)$ to the odds of an insect exposed to a dose (I, S). Because the parameter θ_3 is nonnull, this ratio depends on I:

$$\psi(I; \theta_2, \theta_3) = \exp\left\{\theta_2 \log\left(\frac{2I - \theta_3}{I - \theta_3}\right)\right\}.$$

For several values of I, we can estimate the effect of doubling the dose of insecticide and calculate a confidence interval.

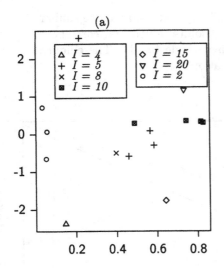
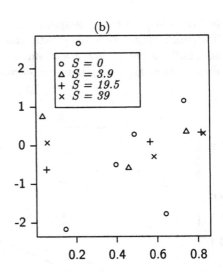

Figure 6.3. Assay of an insecticide with a synergist: Deviance residuals (a) and Pearson residuals (b) versus the fitted probabilities.

Confidence Interval for $\psi(I; \theta_2, \theta_3)$ Based on the Wald Test Because ψ is a positive quantity, it is generally preferable to calculating a confidence interval for $\log(\psi(I; \theta_2, \theta_3))$. In the first step, we calculate $\widehat{I}_N(I)$, the 95% confidence interval for $\log(\psi(I; \theta_2, \theta_3))$, using the method described in Sections 3.4.1 and 3.4.4. Then we take the exponential of each bound of $\widehat{I}_N(I)$ to get a 95% confidence interval for $\psi(I; \theta_2, \theta_3)$.

Results We denote by $\log(\widehat{\psi}(I))$ the estimated value of $\log(\psi(I))$ and by $\widehat{S}(I)$ its estimated standard error. The 95% confidence interval for $\psi(I)$ is denoted by $\exp\left(\widehat{I}_N(I)\right)$:

I	$\log(\widehat{\psi}(I))$	$\widehat{S}(I)$	$\widehat{I}_N(I)$	$\widehat{\psi}(I)$	$\exp\left(\widehat{I}_N\right)$
2	2.64	0.276	[2.09, 3.18]	14.04	[8.16, 24.1]
4	1.34	0.078	[1.19, 1.49]	3.84	[3.29, 4.47]
5	1.23	0.077	[1.08, 1.38]	3.43	[2.95, 3.99]
8	1.09	0.076	[0.95, 1.24]	3.00	[2.58, 3.48]
10	1.06	0.075	[0.91, 1.20]	2.88	[2.49, 3.34]
15	1.01	0.074	[0.86, 1.16]	2.75	[2.38, 3.19]
20	0.99	0.074	[0.84, 1.13]	2.69	[2.33, 3.11]

We have represented the results in Figure 6.4. It appears that for large doses, greater than 8, the effect of doubling the dose of insecticide is to increase the odds of an insect dying by a factor approximatively equal to 2.8.

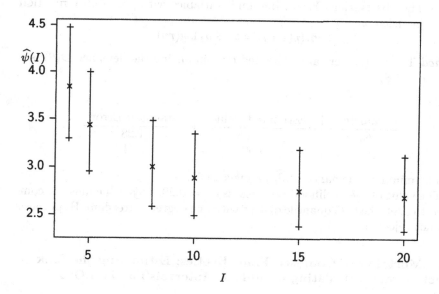

Figure 6.4. Assay of an insecticide with a synergist: Estimated odds ratio when doubling the dose of insecticide for several values of I

6.6.2 Vaso-Constriction in the Skin of the Digits: Estimation and Test of Nested Models

Model The observations Y_i are Bernoulli variables with probability function $p(x, \theta)$ modeled as

$$\left.\begin{aligned} p(x, \theta) &= \exp(\eta(x, \theta))/ \left\{1 + \exp(\eta(x, \theta))\right\}, \\ \eta(x, \theta) &= \theta_0 + \theta_1 \log(r) + \theta_2 \log(v) \end{aligned}\right\}. \quad (6.16)$$

Method The parameters are estimated by minimizing the deviance $D(\theta)$; see Equation (6.8).

Results

Parameters	Estimated Values	Standard Error
θ_0	-2.87	1.32
θ_1	5.18	1.86
θ_2	4.56	1.84

The minimum deviance $D(\widehat{\theta})$ equals 29.23.

Because the estimated values of θ_1 and θ_2 are close together, we want to test the hypothesis H that $\theta_1 = \theta_2$ against the alternative A that $\theta_1 \neq \theta_2$. For using the likelihood ratio test, we have to compare $D(\widehat{\theta})$, the minimum deviance under A, to the minimum deviance under H.

Model The observations Y_i are Bernoulli variables with probability function $p(x, \theta)$ modeled as
$$\text{logit}(p(x, \theta)) = \theta_0 + \theta_3 \log(rv).$$

Method The parameters are estimated by minimizing the deviance $D(\theta)$; see Equation (6.8).

Results

Parameters	Estimated Values	Standard Error
θ_0	-3.03	1.28
θ_3	4.90	1.74

The minimum deviance $D(\widehat{\theta}_{\text{H}})$ equals 29.52.

The value of the likelihood ratio test is $\mathcal{S}_{\text{L}} = 0.29$. This value must be compared to 3.84, the 0.95 quantile of a χ^2 with one degree of freedom. Hypothesis H is not rejected.

6.6.3 Mortality of Confused Flour Beetles: Estimating the Link Function and Calculating Confidence Intervals for the LD90

Model The observations Y_{ij} are binomial variables with probability function $p(x, \theta)$ modeled as

$$\left. \begin{array}{l} p(x, \theta) = 1 - (1 + \theta_3 \exp(\eta(x, \theta)))^{-1/\theta_3} , \\ \eta(x, \theta) = \theta_1 + \theta_2 \log(x) \end{array} \right\}. \qquad (6.17)$$

The definition of the model is complete if we assume that the parameters satisfy the following condition:

$$1 + \theta_3 \exp(\eta(x, \theta)) > 0. \qquad (6.18)$$

If we assume that θ_3 is positive, clearly the condition is always fulfilled no matter the values of x, θ_1, and θ_2.

Method The parameters are estimated by minimizing the deviance $D(\theta)$; see Equation (6.8).

Results

Parameters	Estimated Values	Standard Error
θ_1	-10.78	1.75
θ_2	0.174	0.031
θ_3	0.186	0.279

We notice that the estimated standard error for parameter θ_3 is large compared with the value of θ_3, leading us to suspect that θ_3 is not significantly different from 0.

Testing Nested Models Let us compare this model with two particular nested models. The first one corresponds to the model using the logit link function when $\theta_3 = 1$, and the second one to the model using the cloglog link function when $\theta_3 = 0$.

Model We consider the following two models:

$$p(x, \theta) = \frac{\exp(\eta(x, \theta))}{1 + \exp(\eta(x, \theta))}, \tag{6.19}$$

based on the logit link model, and

$$p(x, \theta) = 1 - \exp\left(-\exp(\eta(x, \theta))\right), \tag{6.20}$$

based on the cloglog link model. The function $\eta(x, \theta)$ is linear in $\log(x)$ (see Equation (6.17)).

Method The parameters are estimated by minimizing the deviance $D(\theta)$; see Equation (6.8).

Results Under the hypothesis that the link function is the logit function, we get the following results:

Parameters	Estimated Values	Standard Error
θ_1	−14.81	1.29
θ_2	0.249	0.021

Under the hypothesis that the link function is the cloglog function, we get

Parameters	Estimated Values	Standard Error
θ_1	−9.75	0.82
θ_2	0.155	0.013

To compare the models defined by Equations (6.17), (6.19), and (6.20), we use the likelihood ratio test described in Section 6.5 for nested models. The values of the minimum deviance are:

	Model (6.17)	Model (6.19)	Model (6.20)
Deviance : $D(\hat{\theta})$	8.19	12.5	8.37

The test statistic for testing that the model is defined by Equation (6.19) against that the model is defined by Equation (6.17) equals 4.31, which must be compared to 3.84, the value of the 0.95 quantile of a χ^2 with one degree of freedom. We thus conclude that the model based on the logit link function is rejected. In contrast, there is no reason to reject the model based on the cloglog link function because the difference in the deviance functions equals 0.18, which is smaller than 3.84. Therefore, to calculate a confidence interval for the LD90, we will consider model (6.20).

Confidence Interval Based on the Likelihood Ratio Test The LD90 is defined as the dose of CS_2 such that the probability of a beetle dying equals 0.9. Namely, considering model (6.20), the LD90 is defined as follows:

$$LD90 = \frac{\log\left(-\log(0.1)\right) - \theta_1}{\theta_2}.$$

To calculate a confidence interval using the likelihood ratio test statistic, we have to introduce LD90 into the model of the probability function $p(x, \theta)$ as a parameter to estimate.

Model Doing so, we get the following model:

$$\text{cloglog}\left(p(x, LD90, \theta_2)\right) = \log(-\log(0.1)) - \theta_2 \log\left(\frac{x}{LD90}\right). \tag{6.21}$$

Result

Parameters	Estimated Values	Standard Error
LD90	68.11	0.705
θ_2	9.57	0.78

As explained in Section 3.5.1, we calculate a 95% confidence interval for LD90 by calculating the set of values ℓ such that the likelihood ratio test at level 5% of hypothesis H_ℓ: LD90 $= \ell$, against the alternative A that there is no constraint on the parameters is not rejected.

For each ℓ, the test statistic equals the difference between $D_\ell = D(\widehat{\theta}_{H_\ell})$, the minimum deviance under the constraint H_ℓ, and $D(\widehat{\theta}) = 8.37$ the minimum deviance under the alternative A. Hypothesis H_ℓ is rejected if $D_\ell - D(\widehat{\theta})$ is greater than 3.84. The variations of $D_\ell - D(\widehat{\theta})$ versus ℓ are shown in Figure 6.5. The horizontal line represents the threshold value equal to 3.84. The estimated confidence interval with level 95% equals [66.8; 69.6] and is represented by the two vertical segments.

6.6.4 Mortality of Confused Flour Beetles 2: Comparison of Curves and Confidence Intervals for the ED50

Model The observations Y_{ij} are binomial variables with probability function $p(x, t, \theta)$ modeled as

$$\left.\begin{aligned} p(x, t, \theta) &= H(x, t, \theta) - H(x, t-1, \theta), \\ H(x, t, \theta) &= (1 + \exp(-\theta_1 - \theta_2 \log(x)))^{-1}(1 + \exp(\theta_3 - \theta_4 \log(t)))^{-1} \end{aligned}\right\}. \tag{6.22}$$

Method The parameters are estimated by minimizing the deviance $D(\theta)$; see Equation (6.8).

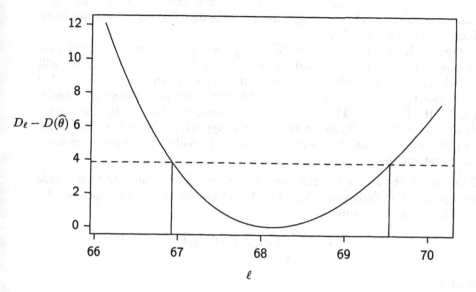

Figure 6.5. Beetles example: Values of the deviance test statistic $D_\ell - D(\widehat{\theta})$ when the parameter LD90 equals ℓ

Results Under the hypothesis that the link function is the logit function, we get the following results:

Parameters	Estimated Values	Standard Error
θ_1^M	5.10	1.48
θ_2^M	3.68	0.97
θ_3^M	2.69	0.22
θ_4^M	2.70	0.19
θ_1^F	2.47	0.66
θ_2^F	2.50	0.48
θ_3^F	4.03	0.35
θ_4^F	3.47	0.28

The minimum deviance $D(\widehat{\theta})$ equals 102.65.

Making Comparisons Fitting the same model to both male and female data sets produced a deviance of 129.13. The likelihood ratio test statistic of the hypothesis that θ does not vary with gender is then $129.13 - 102.65 = 26.48$, to be compared to the quantile of a χ^2 distribution on four degrees of freedom. The hypothesis is rejected.

We can investigate the difference further by assuming that only (θ_1, θ_2) does not vary with gender. The residual deviance is then 117.41, showing a significant effect of gender on (θ_1, θ_2).

Conversely, if we assume that only (θ_3, θ_4) does not vary with gender, the residual deviance is 114.60, suggesting that the distribution of time to death differs between the genders.

Frequently one might expect $\theta_2^M = \theta_2^F$, which is commonly called *parallelism* if the survival distributions are identical. In this example, we will test whether the two logistic nonlinear curves can be taken to be comparable by computing the likelihood ratio test statistic of the parallelism hypothesis: $103.99 - 102.65 = 1.34$. This number must be compared to 3.84, the 0.95 quantile of a χ^2 with one degree of freedom; the hypothesis is not rejected. Then the mean effective dose ED50 may be used to provide a comparison between males and females.

Estimates of the ED50 We can compute an estimate of the ED50, the dose corresponding to 50% mortality. The ED50 for day $t = 13$ is obtained by solving the following equation:

$$0.5 = \sum_{k \leq 13} p(\log(ED50), t_k, \widehat{\theta}),$$

which yields

$$\log(\widehat{ED50}) = -\frac{1}{\widehat{\theta}_2}(\widehat{\theta}_1 + \log(2\widehat{F}(t_{13}) - 1)), \tag{6.23}$$

where $\widehat{F}(t) = (1 + \exp(\widehat{\theta}_3 - \widehat{\theta}_4 \log(t)))^{-1}$.

Confidence Interval for $\log(ED50)$ *Based on the Wald Test*

	$\log \widehat{ED50}$	Standard Error	$\widehat{I}_{\mathcal{N}}$
Males	−1.34	0.068	[−1.477, −1.210]
Females	−1.023	0.078	[−1.176, −0.870]

The ratio of the two effective doses, $\rho = ED50^F/ED50^M$, is termed the susceptibility ratio. We can calculate a Wald-type confidence interval of the susceptibility ratio:

$\widehat{\rho}$	Standard Error	$\widehat{I}_{\mathcal{N}}$
1.38	0.13	[1.15, 1.65]

The interval does not contain 1; males are more susceptible to the insecticide as they have a lower ED50.

Confidence Interval for $\log(ED50)$ *Based on the Likelihood Ratio Test* To calculate a confidence interval using the likelihood ratio test statistic, we have to introduce $ED50$ into the modeling of $p(x, t, \theta)$ as a parameter to estimate.

Model

$$\left. \begin{array}{l} p(x, t, \theta) = H(x, t, \theta) - H(x, t - 1, \theta), \\ H(x, t, \theta) = F(t) \{1 + (2F(t_{13}) - 1) \exp(-\theta_2 \log(x/ED50))\}^{-1} \end{array} \right\}, \tag{6.24}$$

where $F(t) = (1 + \exp(\theta_3 - \theta_4 \log(t)))^{-1}$.

Result

Parameters	Estimated Values	Standard Error
$\log ED50^M$	-1.34	0.07
θ_2^M	2.82	0.43
θ_3^M	2.70	0.22
θ_4^M	2.72	0.19
$\log ED50^F$	-1.02	0.08
θ_2^F	2.82	0.43
θ_3^F	4.02	0.35
θ_4^F	3.46	0.28

The likelihood ratio interval with level 95% equals $[-1.474 - 1.208]$ for the males and $[-1.171 - 0.851]$ for the females.

6.6.5 Germination of Orobranche: Estimating Overdispersion Using the Quasi-Likelihood Estimation Method

Let us estimate the parameters under the binomial linear model.

Model The observations are binomial variables, $Y_{ij} \sim \mathcal{B}(N_{ij}, p(x_i, \theta))$, where $x_i = (S_i, E_i)$ and the probability function is as

$$\text{logit}\,(p(S_i, E_i, \theta)) = \theta_0 + \theta_1 S_i + \theta_2 E_i + \theta_3 S_i E_i. \qquad (6.25)$$

Method The parameters are estimated by minimizing the deviance $D(\theta)$; see Equation (6.8).

Results

Parameters	Estimated Values	Standard Error
θ_0	-0.558	0.126
θ_1	0.146	0.223
θ_2	1.318	0.177
θ_3	-0.778	0.306

Goodness-of-Fit Test As already noted in Section 6.1.5, the model defined by Equation (6.25) corresponds to the saturated model in a 2×2 factorial experiment. Because for each modality of the explanatory variables $x_i = (S_i, E_i)$, we have several replications, we can test hypothesis H that this model is correct against alternative A that the observations are binomial variables with parameters (N_{ij}, p_{ij}). Under A, the p_{ij} are estimated as the empirical frequencies $\pi_{ij} = Y_{ij}/N_{ij}$. We apply the goodness-of-fit test described in Section 6.5 though some of the N_{ij}s are small. The minimum deviance under hypothesis H, $D(\widehat{\theta})$, equals 33.27. This value must be compared to 27.59, the value of the 0.95 quantile of a χ^2 with 17 degrees of freedom. We conclude by rejecting hypothesis H. Because it is not possible to improve the model defined by Equation (6.25), we conclude that the data are overdispersed, and we present the parameter estimation under various modelings of the variance function.

Modeling the Variance Function First we consider the case where the variance function is proportional to the variance of a binomial variable.

Model The observations Y_{ij} satisfy the following two equations:

$$\left. \begin{array}{l} \mathrm{E}(Y_{ij}) = N_{ij}p(x_i,\theta), \\ \mathrm{Var}(Y_{ij}) = \sigma^2 N_{ij}p(x_i,\theta)\left(1 - p(x_i,\theta)\right) \end{array} \right\}, \tag{6.26}$$

where $p(x_i,\theta)$ is defined by Equation (6.25).

Method The estimation of the parameters θ is done as in the binomial case. The parameter σ^2 is estimated by the residual variance; see Equation (6.11).

Result The residual variance $\hat{\sigma}^2$ equals 1.51. The estimated standard errors for the parameters θ are obtained by multiplying the estimated standard errors under the binomial model by $\hat{\sigma}$:

Parameters	Estimated Values	Standard Error
θ_0	−0.558	0.155
θ_1	0.146	0.234
θ_2	1.318	0.218
θ_3	−0.778	0.376

Secondly, we consider the cases where the variability in the probability function is modeled.

Model The observations Y_{ij} satisfy the following two equations:

$$\left. \begin{array}{l} \mathrm{E}(Y_{ij}) = N_{ij}p(x_i,\theta), \\ \mathrm{Var}(Y_{ij}) = N_{ij}p(x_i,\theta)\left(1 - p(x_i,\theta)\right)\left[1 + \tau(N_{ij} - 1)\right] \end{array} \right\}, \tag{6.27}$$

where $p(x_i,\theta)$ is defined by Equation (6.25). When $N_{ij} = N$ for all $i = 1,\ldots,k$ and $j = 1,\ldots,n_i$, this model is the same as the preceding model.

Method The parameters θ and τ are estimated using the quasi-likelihood method described in Section 6.4.2.

Results

Parameters	Estimated Values	Standard Error
θ_0	−0.541	0.164
θ_1	0.096	0.223
θ_2	1.320	0.177
θ_3	−0.798	0.306
τ	0.0126	0.012

The following model is based on the assumption that the observations are distributed as a beta-binomial variable.

Model The observations Y_{ij} satisfy the following two equations:

$$\left. \begin{array}{l} \mathrm{E}(Y_{ij}) = N_{ij}p(x_i,\theta), \\ \mathrm{Var}(Y_{ij}) = N_{ij}p(x_i,\theta)\left(1 - p(x_i,\theta)\right)\left[1 + \tau_i(N_{ij} - 1)\right] \end{array} \right\}, \tag{6.28}$$

where $p(x_i,\theta)$ is defined by Equation (6.25).

Method The parameters θ and $\tau = (\tau_1, \ldots, \tau_k)$ are estimated using the quasi-likelihood method described in Section 6.4.2.

Results

Parameters	Estimated Values	Standard Error
θ_0	-0.538	0.177
θ_1	0.087	0.286
θ_2	1.314	0.239
θ_3	-0.743	0.371
τ_1	0.0177	0.023
τ_2	0.0102	0.017
τ_3	0.0161	0.035
τ_4	0.0016	0.021

Finally, we consider the model based on the assumption that the linear predictor is a Gaussian random variable.

Model The observations Y_{ij} satisfy the following two equations:

$$\left.\begin{array}{l} \mathrm{E}(Y_{ij}) = N_{ij}p(x_i, \theta), \\ \mathrm{Var}(Y_{ij}) = N_{ij}p(x_i, \theta)\left(1 - p(x_i, \theta)\right)\left[1 + \tau(N_{ij} - 1)p(x_i, \theta)\left(1 - p(x_i, \theta)\right)\right] \end{array}\right\},$$
$$(6.29)$$

where $p(x_i, \theta)$ is defined by Equation (6.25).

Method The parameters θ and τ are estimated using the quasi-likelihood method described in Section 6.4.2.

Results

Parameters	Estimated Values	Standard Error
θ_0	-0.540	0.164
θ_1	0.095	0.273
θ_2	1.319	0.234
θ_3	-0.800	0.380
τ	0.055	0.051

Confidence Interval for the Parameter of Overdispersion

Looking at the results, the overdispersion does not seem to be significant in this data set. To appreciate if this is indeed the case, let us calculate a confidence interval for τ in the model defined by Equation (6.27).

Calculation of a Confidence Interval for τ Using the Wald Statistic

Standard calculations lead to the following result:

$\hat{\tau}$	$\hat{S}$	$\nu_{0.975}$	$\hat{I}_{\mathcal{N}}$
0.0126	0.0117	1.96	$[-0.0103, 0.0355]$

Calculation of a Confidence Interval for τ Using the Bootstrap Method

We calculate a bootstrap confidence interval for τ exactly as we did in Section 3.5.1 for the parameter θ_3.

We get the following result, based on $B = 500$ bootstrap simulations:

$\widehat{\tau}$	$\widehat{S}$	$b_{0.025}$	$b_{0.975}$	$\widehat{I}_B$
0.0126	0.0117	−4.225	0.815	[0.00305, 0.0621]

The bootstrap interval does not contain 0, while the confidence interval based on the Wald test does contain 0. We are thus led to conclude that the overdispersion is light but significant.

6.7 Using nls2

This section reproduces the commands and files used in this chapter to analyze the examples using **nls2**. For each example, we first create the *data frame* to store the experimental data, then we estimate the parameters using the quasi-likelihood method.

Assay of an Insecticide with a Synergist

Creating the Data

The experimental data (see Table 6.1, page 154) are stored in a *data frame* called `insect`:

```
> y <- c(7, 59, 115, 149, 178, 229, 5, 43, 76, 4, 57, 83, 6, 57, 84)
> n <- c(100, 200, rep(300,4), rep(100,9))
> DI <- c(4, 5, 8, 10, 15, 20, 2, 5, 10, 2, 5, 10, 2, 5, 10)
> DS <- c(rep(0,6), rep(3.9,3), rep(19.5,3), rep(39,3))
> insect <- data.frame(y=y,n=n,DI=DI,DS=DS)
```

Parameter Estimation by Minimizing the Deviance Function

We describe the model given by Equation (6.14), page 167, in a file called `insect.m`:

```
% file insect.m
% logistic non-linear regression model
% with binomial distribution
resp y;
var v;
varind DI,DS,n;
aux eta,p;
parresp t1,t2,t3,t4,t5;
subroutine;
```

```
begin
eta = t1+t2*log(DI-t3)+t4*DS/(t5+DS);
p=exp(eta)/(1+exp(eta));
y = n*p;
v = n*(1-p)*p;
end
```

To find reasonable starting values for the parameters, we make a binomial linear regression using the function glm in S-Plus. Namely, we model the linear predictor η as follows:

$$\eta(x, \theta) = \beta_1 + \beta_2 \log(I) + \beta_3 S.$$

```
> insect.glm <- glm(formula  = cbind(y,n-y) ~ log(DI) + DS,
                     family=binomial)
```

Then we call **nls2** using its arguments as follows:

- The argument **method**—because minimizing the deviance $D(\theta)$ is equivalent to solving the quasi-likelihood equations, we will use **nls2** by setting the argument **method** to the value **"QLT"**.
- The argument **stat.ctx**—it should be noted that in a binomial model, the variance function can be written as follows:

$$\text{var}(Y_{ij}) = \sigma^2 g(x_i, N_{ij}; \theta, \tau)$$

with $\sigma^2 = 1$ and $g(x_i, N_{ij}; \theta, \tau) = N_{ij} p(x_i, \theta)(1 - p(x_i, \theta))$. Therefore we have to use the components **sigma2.type** and **sigma2** of the argument **stat.ctx** that describes the statistical context of the analysis. By setting **sigma2.type** to the value **"KNOWN"** and **sigma2** to the value 1, we specify that σ^2 is known and equal to 1. Therefore σ^2 will not be estimated by the residual variance, but will stay fixed to the value 1 throughout the estimation process.

  Moreover, the calculations of the maximum likelihood, the minimum deviance, and the deviance residuals will be done only if the component **family** is set to the value **"binomial"** and if the component **nameN** contains the name of the variable N in the *data frame* containing the data.

- The argument **model**—the model defined by Equation (6.14) implicitly assumes that the parameter θ_3 is smaller than 2, the smallest value of the dose of insecticide, and that the parameter θ_5 is positive. These constraints on the parameters are specified using the components **sup.theta** and **inf.theta** of the argument **model**:

```
> ctx <- list(theta.start=c(insect.glm$coeff[1:2],0,
                            insect.glm$coeff[3],1),
              sigma2.type="KNOWN", sigma2=1,
              family="binomial", nameN="n")
> mod <- list(file="insect.m",
```

```
              sup.theta=c(NaN,NaN,2,NaN,NaN),
              inf.theta=c(NaN,NaN,NaN,NaN,0))
> insect.nl1 <- nls2( insect, mod, stat.ctx=ctx, method="QLT")
```

Then we display the result of the estimation process (see page 168):

```
> cat( "Result of the estimation process:\n ")
> print(summary(insect.nl1))
```

The logarithm of the likelihood for binomial data and the minimum deviance (see Equation (6.8) and Section 6.4.1) are given, respectively, by the components log.binomial and deviance of the output argument of nls2. Besides, the deviance residuals defined by Equation (6.15) and the Pearson residuals are given by the components dev.residuals and s.residuals. The X^2 of Pearson defined as $X^2 = \sum_{i=1}^{k} \sum_{j=1}^{n_i} (\hat{e}_{ij})^2$ is the residual sum of squares and is given by the component rss:

```
> cat( "\nValue of the log-likelihood:\n ")
> print(insect.nl1$log.binomial)
> cat( "\nvalue of the minimum deviance:\n ")
> print(insect.nl1$deviance)
> cat( "\nDeviance residuals:\n ")
> print(insect.nl1$dev.residuals)
> cat( "\nvalue of the X2 of Pearson:\n ")
> print(insect.nl1$rss)
> cat( "\nPearson residuals:\n ")
> print(insect.nl1$s.residuals)
```

Graphics for Diagnostic

The graphics of fitted probabilities versus the observed frequencies and the graphics of residuals are done using the plot functions of S-Plus (see Figures 6.2 and 6.3):

```
> freq <- insect$y/insect$n
> proba <- insect.nl1$response/insect$n
> plot( proba, freq, las=1,
    xlab="observed frequency",ylab="fitted probability")
> abline(0,1)
> par(mfrow=c(1,2))
> plot( proba, insect.nl1$dev.residuals,
    ylab="deviance residuals", xlab="fitted probability",
    type="n")
> text( proba, insect.nl1$dev.residuals,
    labels=insect$DI)
> plot( proba, insect.nl1$s.residuals,
    ylab="Pearson residuals", xlab="fitted probability",
    type="n")
> text( proba, insect.nl1$s.residuals,
    labels=insect$DS)
```

Confidence Interval for $\log(\psi(I))$ *Based on the Wald Test*

For each value of I, we calculate the confidence interval $\widehat{I}_N$ using the function **confidence**. We display the estimated values of $\log(\psi(I))$ and $\widehat{I}_N$ (see page 169).

First, the function $\log(\psi(I))$ is described in a file called **oddsRatio.m**:

```
% file oddsRatio.m
% log-odds ratio as function of I
psi logpsi;
ppsi t2,t3;
varpsi I;
subroutine;
begin
logpsi=t2*log((2*I-t3)/(I-t3));
end
```

Then we apply the function **confidence** and display the results:

```
> I <- sort(unique(DI))
> loadnls2(psi="")
> ConfInt.logPsi <- confidence.nls2( insect.nl1, file="oddsRatio.m",
                  varpsi = I)
> Int <- cbind(ConfInt.logPsi$psi, ConfInt.logPsi$normal.conf.int)
> cat("Estimated values of the log odds ratio:\n")
> print(cbind(I,Int[,1]))
> cat("95% Confidence Interval for the log odds ratio:\n")
> print(Int[,2:3])
```

Finally, we get a confidence interval for $\psi(I)$, taking the exponential of the confidence interval for $\log(\psi(I))$:

```
> Int <- cbind(I,exp(Int))
> dimnames(Int) <- list(NULL,c("I","Psi","Inf.Psi","Sup.Psi"))
> cat("Estimated values of the odds ratio:\n")
> cat("and Confidence Interval:\n")
> print(Int)
```

Vaso-Constriction in the Skin of the Digits

Binary data are treated in the same way as binomial data. Because for all i and j, $N_{ij} = 1$, the values of the N_{ij}s are not required.

Creating the Data

The experimental data (see Table 6.2, page 155) are stored in a *data frame* called **vaso**:

```
> vol <- c(
    3.70, 0.80, 0.90, 0.60, 3.20, 0.40, 1.60, 1.90, 1.10,
    0.95, 3.50, 0.70, 0.90, 1.40, 0.85, 0.95, 0.60, 1.60,
```

```
      1.10, 0.75, 1.25, 0.60, 0.80, 0.75, 1.70, 1.35, 1.80,
      2.70, 1.20, 1.30, 0.75, 1.10, 0.55, 2.30, 1.80, 1.50,
      0.95, 2.35, 0.80)
> rate <- c(
      0.825, 3.200, 0.750, 3.000, 1.600, 2.000, 1.780, 0.950,
      1.830, 1.900, 1.090, 3.500, 0.450, 2.330, 1.415, 1.360,
      1.500, 0.400, 2.200, 1.900, 2.500, 0.750, 0.570, 3.750,
      1.060, 1.350, 1.500, 0.750, 2.000, 1.625, 1.500, 1.700,
      2.750, 1.640, 1.800, 1.360, 1.900, 0.030, 3.330)
> y <- c(
      1, 1, 0, 0, 1, 0, 1, 1, 0, 0, 1, 1, 0, 1, 1, 0, 0, 0, 1,
      0, 1, 0, 0, 1, 0, 0, 1, 1, 1, 1, 1, 0, 0, 1, 1, 0, 0, 0,1)
> vaso <- data.frame(vol=vol,rate=rate,y=y)
```

Description of the Model

The linear logistic regression model defined in Equation (6.16), page 171, is described in a file called vaso.m:

```
% file vaso.m
% linear logistic regression model
%
resp y;
varind vol,rate;
aux eta,p;
var v;
parresp t0,t1,t2;
subroutine;
begin
eta=t0+t1*log(vol)+t2*log(rate);
p=exp(eta)/(1+exp(eta));
y=p;
v = (1-p)*p;
end
```

Then we call nls2 using the arguments method and stat.ctx as described earlier (see page 181). The component family of the argument stat.ctx is set to the value "bernoulli". We display the estimated values of the parameters, their asymptotic standard errors, and the minimum deviance (see page 171):

```
> ctx <- list(theta.start=rep(0,3), sigma2.type="KNOWN", sigma2=1,
              family="bernoulli")
> vaso.nl1 <- nls2(vaso, "vaso.m", ctx, method="QLT")
> cat( "Result of the estimation process:\n ")
> print(summary(vaso.nl1))
> cat( "\nvalue of the minimum deviance:\n ")
> print(vaso.nl1$deviance)
```

Likelihood Ratio Test of H: $\theta_1 = \theta_2$ Against A: $\theta_1 \neq \theta_2$

We estimate the parameters under the constraint that $\theta_1 = \theta_2$ and calculate the corresponding minimum deviance. Then we display the estimated values of the parameters, their asymptotic standard errors, and the minimum deviance. We display the test statistic S_L (see Equation (6.12), page 167) and the 0.95 quantile of a χ^2 with one degree of freedom with which it should be compared (see page 172):

```
> model <- list(file="vaso.m", eqp.theta=c(1,2,2))
> vaso.nl2 <- nls2(vaso, model, ctx, method="QLT")
> cat( "Result of the estimation process\n ")
> cat( "under the hypothesis A ''t1=t2'':\n ")
> print(summary(vaso.nl2))
> cat( "\nvalue of the minimum deviance\n ")
> cat( "under the hypothesis A ''t1=t2'':\n ")
> print(vaso.nl2$deviance)
> cat( "SL:",
      (vaso.nl2$deviance - vaso.nl1$deviance),
      "X2(0.95,1):",  qchisq(0.95,1), "\n\n")
```

Mortality of Confused Flour Beetles

Creating the Data

The experimental data (see Table 6.3, page 156) are stored in a *data frame* called beetles:

```
> CS2 <- c(
    49.06, 52.99, 56.91, 60.84, 64.76, 68.69, 72.61, 76.54)
> y <- c(
    2, 7, 9, 14, 23, 29, 29, 29, 4, 6, 9, 14, 29, 24, 32, 31)
> n <- c(
    29, 30, 28, 27, 30, 31, 30, 29, 30, 30, 34, 29, 33, 28, 32, 31)
> beetles <- data.frame(CS2=rep(CS2,2), y=y, n=n)
```

Estimating the Link Function

The model defined at Equation (6.17), page 172, is described in a file called beetles.m:

```
%   file beetles.m
%   General link function
resp y;
varind CS2,n;
aux p, eta;
var v;
parresp t1,t2,t3;
subroutine;
```

```
begin
eta = t1 + t2*CS2;
p = 1-exp(-(log(1+t3*exp(eta))/t3));
y = n*p;
v = n*(1-p)*p;
end
```

We estimate the parameters using nls2, as described at page 181, for the example with insecticide and synergists. We first estimate the parameters under the constraint that $\theta_3 = 1$ using the component eq.theta of the argument model. Then we estimate the parameters without any constraint on θ_3. We display the parameters and the corresponding minimum deviance (see page 172):

```
> ctx <- list(theta.start=c(0,0,1), sigma2.type="KNOWN", sigma2=1,
>             family="binomial", nameN="n"))
> model <- list(file="beetles.m",eq.theta=c(NaN,NaN,1))
> beetles.nl1 <- nls2(beetles, model,ctx,method="QLT")
> cat( "\nResult of the estimation process:\n ")
> print(summary(beetles.nl1))
> cat( "\nvalue of the minimum deviance:\n ")
> print(beetles.nl1$deviance)
> ctx$theta.start <- beetles.nl1$theta
> beetles.nl2 <- nls2(beetles, "beetles.m", ctx, method="QLT")
> cat( ":\nLogit model:\n")
> cat( "Result of the estimation process:\n")
> print(summary(beetles.nl2))
> cat( "\nvalue of the minimum deviance:\n ")
> print(beetles.nl2$deviance)
```

Testing Nested Models

Though the cloglog model is nested in the general model defined by Equation (6.17), it cannot be described by the constraint $\theta_3 = 0$. Therefore it is necessary to use the file called beetles.mw to describe it:

```
% file beetles.mw
% weibull  regression model
resp y;
varind CS2,n;
aux p, eta;
var v;
parresp t1,t2;
subroutine;
begin
eta = t1 + t2* CS2;
p=1-exp(-exp(eta));
y = n*p;
v = n*(1-p)*p;
end
```

We estimate and display the parameters and the corresponding minimum deviance (see page 173):

```
> ctx$theta.start <- c(0,0)
> beetles.nl3 <- nls2(beetles, "beetles.mw",ctx,method="QLT")
> cat( ":\ncloglog model:\n")
> cat( "Result of the estimation process:\n")
> print(summary(beetles.nl3))
> cat( "\nvalue of the minimum deviance:\n ")
> print(beetles.nl3$deviance)
```

We calculate and display the test statistic S_L (see Equation (6.12), page 167) for each hypothesis we want to test: first to test that the model is the logit model and second to test that the model is the cloglog model. The 0.95 quantile of a χ^2 with one degree of freedom, with which it should be compared, is displayed:

```
> cat( "\nvalue of the minimum deviance\n ")
> cat( "under the general hypothesis:\n ")
> print(beetles.nl1$deviance)
> cat( "\nvalue of the minimum deviance\n ")
> cat( "under the logit hypothesis:\n ")
> print(beetles.nl2$deviance)
> cat( "SL:",
       (beetles.nl1$deviance - beetles.nl2$deviance),
       "X2(0.95,1):",  qchisq(0.95,1), "\n\n")
> cat( "\nvalue of the minimum deviance\n ")
> cat( "under the cloglog hypothesis:\n ")
> print(beetles.nl3$deviance)
> cat( "SL:",
       (beetles.nl1$deviance - beetles.nl3$deviance),
       "X2(0.95,1):",  qchisq(0.95,1), "\n\n")
```

Confidence Interval for the LD90

To calculate the confidence interval based on the log-likelihood ratio, first we have to plug the LD90 into the cloglog model as a parameter to estimate (see Equation (6.21), page 174). The file called **beetles.mLD90** describes the new parameterization of the cloglog model:

```
% file beetles.mLD90
% weibull regression model
% new parametrisation : t2, LD90
resp y;
varind CS2,n;
aux p, eta;
var v;
parresp LD90,t2;
subroutine;
```

```
begin
eta = log(-log(0.1))+ t2* (CS2 - LD90);
p=1-exp(-exp(eta));
y = n*p;
v = n*(1-p)*p;
end
```

Then we carry out the calculations done on page 174 and shown in Figure 6.5. The function conflike dealing with Gaussian errors cannot be used for binomial likelihood:

```
> ctx$theta.start <- c(70,0.2)
> beetles.nl4 <- nls2(beetles, "beetles.mLD90", ctx, method="QLT")
> LD90 <- beetles.nl4$theta[1]
> cat("Estimated value of LD90:", LD90,"\n" )
> cat("Estimated value of S:",
        summary(beetles.nl4)$std.error[1],"\n")
> se.LD90 <- summary(beetles.nl4)$std.error[1]
> grid <- seq(LD90-3*se.LD90,LD90+3*se.LD90,length=50)
> Diff <- rep(0,length(grid))
> for (l in 1:length(grid)) {
>    ctx$theta.start <- c(grid[l],beetles.nl4$theta[2])
>    model <- list(file="beetles.mLD90", eq.theta=c(grid[l],NaN))
>    Diff[l] <- nls2(beetles, model, ctx, method="QLT")$deviance
> }
> ind1 <- 1:(length(grid)/2)
> ind2 <- (length(grid)/2):length(grid)
> LD90Inf <- approx( Diff[ind1]-beetles.nl3$deviance,
                    grid[ind1], xout=3.84)$y
> LD90Sup <- approx( Diff[ind2]-beetles.nl3$deviance,
                    grid[ind2],xout=3.84)$y
> cat("\n95% Confidence Interval:\n",
> print(cbind(LD90Inf,LD90,LD90Sup))
```

Mortality of Confused Flour Beetles 2

Creating the Data The experimental data (see Table 6.4, page 158) are stored in a *data frame* called fbeetles:

```
> dose <- c(rep(0.2,13), rep(0.32,13), rep(0.5,13), rep(0.8,13))
> tps <- rep(1:13,4)
> curves <- c(rep("M",52), rep("F",52))
> y <- c(3, 11, 10, 7, 4, 3, 2, 1, 0, 0, 0, 1, 1,
          7, 10, 11,16, 3, 2, 1, rep(0,6),
          5,  8, 11,15, 4, 2, 1, 1, rep(0,5),
          4, 10,  8,14, 8, 2, 1, 0, 0, 1, 0, 0, 0,
          0,  2,  4, 8, 9, 3, rep(0,7),
          1,  5, 11,10, 5, 1, 0, 1, rep(0,5),
          0,  4,  6, 6, 3, 1, 1, 4, 0, 0, 0, 1, 1,
```

```
              2,  7, 15, 9, 3, 4, 1, 1, 0, 1, 0, 0, 0)
> n <- c(rep(144,13), rep(69,13), rep(54,13), rep(50,13),
              rep(152,13), rep(81,13), rep(44,13), rep(47,13))
> fbeetles <- data.frame( logd=log(dose),
                             y=y, n=n, tps=tps, curves=curves)
```

Description of the Model The model defined in Equation (6.22), is described in a file called **fbeetles.m**:

```
% file fbeetles.m
resp y;
var v;
varind logd,tps,n;
aux eta,Fplus,Fmoins,p;
parresp t1,t2,t3,t4;
subroutine;
begin
eta = - (t1+t2*logd);
Fplus=1/(1+exp(t3-t4*log(tps)));
Fmoins=  if tps==1 then 0
           else 1/(1+exp(t3-t4*log(tps-1)))
           fi;
p=(Fplus-Fmoins)/(1+exp(eta));
y = n*p;
v = n*(1-p)*p;
end
```

We estimate the parameters using **nls2**, as described at page 181 for the example with insecticide and synergists. The results of the estimation are stored in the structure called **fbeetles.nl1**:

```
> ctx <- list(theta.start=rep(c(4.5,3,2.5,3),2),
              sigma2.type="KNOWN", sigma2=1,
              family="binomial", nameN="n")
> fbeetles.nl1 <- nls2(fbeetles, "fbeetles.m", ctx, method="QLT")
> cat("\n Result of the estimation process: \n")
> print(summary(fbeetles.nl1))
> cat("\n value of the minimum deviance: \n")
> print(fbeetles.nl1$deviance)
```

Comparison of Curves We calculate the likelihood ratio statistics corresponding to each test (see page 175). Estimation under each hypothesis is done by setting equality constraints on a subset of the parameters using the component eqp.theta of the argument model:

```
> model <- list(file="fbeetles.m", eqp.theta=c(1,2,3,4,1,2,3,4))
> fbeetles.nl2 <- nls2(fbeetles, model, ctx, method="QLT")
> model$eqp.theta <- c(1,2,3,4,1,2,5,6)
> fbeetles.nl3 <- nls2(fbeetles, model, ctx, method="QLT")
> model$eqp.theta <- c(1,2,3,4,5,6,3,4)
> fbeetles.nl4 <- nls2(fbeetles, model, ctx, method="QLT")
```

```
> model$eqp.theta <- c(1,2,3,4,5,2,6,7)
> fbeetles.nl5 <- nls2(fbeetles, model, ctx, method="QLT")
```

To test the equality of the two curves, we compare the test statistic to the 0.95 quantile of a χ^2 with four degrees of freedom:

```
> cat("SL:", (fbeetles.nl2$deviance - fbeetles.nl1$deviance),
       "X2(0.95,4):", qchisq(0.95,4),"\n\n")
```

To test the hypothesis that (θ_1, θ_2) does not vary with gender, we compare the test statistic to the 0.95 quantile of a χ^2 with two degrees of freedom:

```
> cat("SL:", (fbeetles.nl3$deviance - fbeetles.nl1$deviance),
       "X2(0.95,2):", qchisq(0.95,2),"\n\n")
```

To test the hypothesis that (θ_3, θ_4) does not vary with gender, we compare the test statistic to the 0.95 quantile of a χ^2 with two degrees of freedom:

```
> cat("SL:", (fbeetles.nl4$deviance - fbeetles.nl1$deviance),
       "X2(0.95,2):", qchisq(0.95,2),"\n\n")
```

To test the hypothesis that $\theta_2^M = \theta_2^F$, we compare the test statistic to the 0.95 quantile of a χ^2 with one degree of freedom:

```
> cat("SL:", (fbeetles.nl5$deviance - fbeetles.nl1$deviance),
       "X2(0.95,1):", qchisq(0.95,1),"\n\n")
```

Wald Confidence Interval for the ED50 We describe $\log ED50^M$ and $\log ED50^F$ as functions of the parameters in two files fED50.mM and fED50.mF (see Equation (6.23) page 176):

```
% file fED50.mM
psi logpsi;
ppsi t1_c1,t2_c1,t3_c1,t4_c1;
varpsi tps;
aux F,X;
subroutine;
begin
F=1/(1+exp(t3_c1-t4_c1*log(tps)));
X=2*F-1;
logpsi= (-t1_c1-log(X))/t2_c1;
end

% file fED50.mF
psi logpsi;
ppsi t1_c2,t2_c1,t3_c2,t4_c2;
varpsi tps;
aux F,X;
subroutine;
begin
F=1/(1+exp(t3_c2-t4_c2*log(tps)));
X=2*F-1;
logpsi= (-t1_c2-log(X))/t2_c1;
end
```

The function `confidence` is applied to the structure `fbeetles.nl5`, which contains the results of estimation under the hypothesis $\theta_2^M = \theta_2^F$, and the confidence intervals for $\log(ED50)$ are displayed:

```
> loadnls2(psi="")
> temps <- unique(fbeetles$tps)
> ED50.conf.13M <- confidence.nls2( fbeetles.nl5,
                    file="fED50.mM", varpsi=temps[13])
> ED50.conf.13F <- confidence.nls2( fbeetles.nl5,
                    file="fED50.mF", varpsi=temps[13])
> cat("\n Estimated value and standard error \n")
> cat(" of the log ED50 for the males: \n")
> print(c(ED50.conf.13M$psi,ED50.conf.13M$std.error))
> cat("95% confidence interval of the log ED50 for the males: \n")
> print(ED50.conf.13M$normal.conf.int)
> cat("\n Estimated value and standard error \n")
> cat("of the log ED50 for the females: \n")
> print(c(ED50.conf.13F$psi,ED50.conf.13F$std.error))
> cat("95% confidence interval of the log ED50 for the females: \n")
> print(ED50.conf.13F$normal.conf.int)
```

Wald Confidence Interval for the Susceptibility Ratio We describe $\log \rho = \log(ED50^F/ED50^M)$ as a function of the parameters in a file `fratio.m`:

```
% file fratio.m
psi logpsi;
ppsi t1_c1,t2_c1,t3_c1,t4_c1,t1_c2,t3_c2,t4_c2;
varpsi tps;
aux FM,XM,FF,XF;
subroutine;
begin
FM=1/(1+exp(t3_c1-t4_c1*log(tps)));
XM=2*FM-1;
FF=1/(1+exp(t3_c2-t4_c2*log(tps)));
XF=2*FF-1;
logpsi= (-t1_c2-log(XF))/t2_c1 + (t1_c1+log(XM))/t2_c1   ;
end
```

Then we apply the function `confidence`:

```
> ratio.conf.13 <- confidence.nls2( fbeetles.nl5,
                  file="fratio.m", varpsi=temps[13])
```

Finally, we obtain a confidence interval for ρ by taking the exponential of the confidence interval for $\log \rho$ (see page 176):

```
> cat("\n Estimated value of the susceptibility ratio \n")
> print(c(exp(ratio.conf.13$psi),
          exp(ratio.conf.13$psi)*ratio.conf.13$std.error))
> cat("95% confidence interval of the susceptibility ratio: \n")
> print(exp(ratio.conf.13$normal.conf.int))
```

Likelihood Ratio Confidence Interval for the ED50 To calculate the confidence intervals based on the log-likelihood ratio, we must first plug the ED50 into the model as a parameter to estimate, according to Equation (6.24) page 176. The file called fbeetles.mED50 describes the model with the new parameterization:

```
% file feetles.mED50
% new parametrisation :  log(ED50), t2, t3, t4
resp y;
var v;
varind logd,tps,n;
aux eta,Fplus,Fmoins,p,F13;
parresp lED,t2,t3,t4;
subroutine;
begin
F13 = 1/(1+exp(t3-t4*log(13)));
eta = - t2*(logd-lED)+log(2*F13-1);
Fplus=1/(1+exp(t3-t4*log(tps)));
Fmoins=  if tps==1 then 0
         else 1/(1+exp(t3-t4*log(tps-1)))
         fi;
p=(Fplus-Fmoins)/(1+exp(eta));
y = n*p;
v = n*(1-p)*p;
end
```

Then we carry out similar calculations, as for Example 6.1.3 when calculating a confidence interval for the LD90 (see page 187) successively for males and females:

```
> ctx$theta.start <- c(-1.5,3,2.5,3),2)
> model <- list(file="fbeetles.mED50", eqp.theta=c(1,2,3,4,5,2,6,7))
> fbeetles.nl6 <- nls2(fbeetles, model, ctx, method="QLT")
> cat("\n Result of the estimation process: \n")
> print(summary(fbeetles.nl6))
>
> ED50M <- fbeetles.nl6$theta[1]
> se.ED50M <- summary(fbeetles.nl6)$std.error[1]
> grid <- seq(ED50M-3*se.ED50M,ED50M+3*se.ED50M,length=50)
> Diff <- rep(0,length(grid))
> for (l in 1:length(grid)) {
>    ctx$theta.start <- c(grid[l],fbeetles.nl6$theta[2:8])
>    model$eq.theta <- c(grid[l],rep(NaN,7))
>    Diff[l] <- nls2(fbeetles, model, ctx, method="QLT")$deviance
> }
> ind1 <- 1:(length(grid)/2)
> ind2 <- (length(grid)/2):length(grid)
> ED50MInf <- approx( Diff[ind1]-fbeetles.nl6$deviance,
                      grid[ind1], xout=3.84)$y
> ED50MSup <- approx( Diff[ind2]-fbeetles.nl6$deviance,
```

```
                          grid[ind2], xout=3.84)$y
> cat("\n Likelihood Confidence interval for ED50M: \n")
> cbind(ED50MInf,ED50M,ED50MSup)
>
> ED50F <- fbeetles.nl6$theta[5]
> se.ED50F <- summary(fbeetles.nl6)$std.error[5]
> grid <- seq(ED50F-3*se.ED50F,ED50F+3*se.ED50F,length=50)
> Diff <- rep(0,length(grid))
> for (l in 1:length(grid)) {
    ctx$theta.start=c(fbeetles.nl6$theta[1:4],grid[l],
                          fbeetles.nl6$theta[6:8])
>   model$eq.theta <- c(rep(NaN,4), grid[l], rep(NaN,3))
>   Diff[l] <- nls2(fbeetles, model, ctx, method="QLT")$deviance
> }
> ind1 <- 1:(length(grid)/2)
> ind2 <- (length(grid)/2):length(grid)
> ED50FInf <- approx( Diff[ind1]-fbeetles.nl6$deviance,
                          grid[ind1], xout=3.84)$y
> ED50FSup <- approx( Diff[ind2]-fbeetles.nl6$deviance,
                          grid[ind2], xout=3.84)$y
> cat("\n Likelihood Confidence interval for ED50F: \n")
> cbind(ED50FInf,ED50F,ED50FSup)
```

Germination of Orobranche

We first create the *data frame* to store the experimental data. Then we estimate the parameters in the binomial linear model described in Equation (6.25) using the function glm in S-Plus.

Creating the Data

The experimental data (see Table 6.5, page 159) are stored in a *data frame* called orobranche:

```
> y <- c(
    10, 23, 23, 26, 17, 5, 53, 55, 32, 46, 10, 8, 10, 8, 23, 0,
    3, 22, 15, 32, 3)
> n <- c(
    39, 62, 81, 51, 39, 6, 74, 72, 51, 79, 13, 16, 30, 28, 45, 4,
    12, 41, 30, 51, 7)
> sp <- c( rep(0,11), rep(1,10))
> ex <- c( rep(0,5), rep(1,6), rep(0,5), rep(1,5))
> orobranche <- data.frame( y=y, n=n, sp=sp, ex=ex)
```

Estimating the Binomial Linear Model

First the data are fitted with the model described in Equation (6.25), page 177, using the function glm in S-Plus. The results of the estimation are displayed, and the minimum deviance is compared with the 0.95 quantile of a χ^2 with 17 degrees of freedom:

```
> orobranche.glm <- glm(cbind(y,n-y) ~ sp*ex,  family=binomial)
> cat("\nEstimated parameters and standard errors:\n")
> print(summary(orobranche.glm)$coef)
> cat("\nvalue of the minimum deviance:", orobranche.glm$deviance,
      "X2(0.95,17):",  qchisq(0.95,17), "\n\n")
```

Introducing the Coefficient σ^2 in the Variance Function

We estimate the parameters in the model described in Equation (6.26) using the function nls2. We describe the model in a file called **orobranche.m1**:

```
% file orobranche.m1
% logistic linear regression model
% binomial variance
resp y;
varind sp,ex,n;
aux eta,p;
var v;
parresp a,b,c,d;
subroutine;
begin
eta=a + b*sp + c*ex + d*sp*ex;
p=exp(eta)/(1+exp(eta));
y = n*p;
v = n*(1-p)*p;
end
```

Then we call nls2 using its arguments as follows.

- The argument **method** is set to the value "QLT".
- Because σ^2 is an unknown parameter that has to be estimated, the components **sigma2.type** and **sigma2** of the argument **stat.ctx** are set to their default values.

The estimated parameters and their standard errors are displayed.

```
> orobranche.nl11 <- nls2(orobranche, "orobranche.m1",
                          rep(0,4), method="QLT")
> cat( "Result of the estimation process:\n ")
> print(summary(orobranche.nl11))
```

Modeling the Variance Function as in Equation (6.27)

The model is described in a file called **orobranche.m2**:

```
% file orobranche.m2
% logistic linear regression model
% overdispersion : one parameter tau
resp y;
varind sp,ex,n;
aux eta,p;
```

```
var v;
parresp a,b,c,d;
parvar tau;
subroutine;
begin
eta=a + b*sp + c*ex + d*sp*ex;
p=exp(eta)/(1+exp(eta));
y = n*p;
v = n*(1-p)*p*(1+(n-1)*tau);
end
```

Then we call **nls2** using its arguments as follows:

- The argument **method**. The parameters θ and τ are estimated by solving the quasi-likelihood equations defined in Section 3.3.2. **nls2** is used by setting the argument **method** to the value **"QLTB"**.
- The variance function can be written as follows:

$$\mathrm{var}(Y_{ij}) = \sigma^2 g(x_i, N_{ij}; \theta, \tau)$$

with $\sigma^2 = 1$. Therefore we have to use the components **sigma2.type** and **sigma2** of the argument **stat.ctx** that describes the statistical context of the analysis. By setting **sigma2.type** to the value **"KNOWN"** and **sigma2** to the value 1, we specify that σ^2 is known and equal to 1. Therefore σ^2 will not be estimated by the residual variance but will stay fixed to the value 1 throughout the estimation process:

```
> ctx <- list(theta.start=orobranche.nl11$theta,
              beta.start=0,
              sigma2.type="KNOWN", sigma2=1)
> orobranche.nl2 <- nls2(orobranche, "orobranche.m2", ctx,
                         method="QLTB")
> cat( "Result of the estimation process:\n ")
> print(summary(orobranche.nl2))
```

Confidence Interval for τ Using the Wald Test

We display the values of $\hat{\tau}$, $\hat{S}$, $\nu_{0.975}$, and $\hat{I}_N$:

```
> tau <- orobranche.nl2$beta
> Stau <- sqrt(orobranche.nl2$as.var[5, 5])
> cat("Estimated value of tau:", tau,"\n" )
> cat("Estimated value of S:", Stau,"\n" )
> cat("nu_(0.975):", qnorm(0.975),"\n" )
> cat("Estimated value of In:",
    c(tau-qnorm(0.975)*Stau,
      tau+qnorm(0.975)*Stau)
    ,"\n" )
```

Confidence Interval for τ Using Bootstrap with Asymptotic Level 95%

To calculate the confidence interval $\widehat{I}_B$ defined in Section 3.4.3, page 71, we use the function **bootstrap**. Several methods of bootstrap simulation are possible. Here, we choose **wild.2**, which means that pseudoerrors are obtained by multiplying the residuals by the independent random variables T defined in Equation (3.15), page 72.

To initialize the iterative process of **bootstrap**, **nls2** must be called with the option **renls2**. We also set the option **control** so that intermediate results are not printed. Finally, we call the function **delnls2** to destroy any internal structures:

```
> orobranche.nl2 <- nls2(orobranche, "orobranche.m2",
               ctx, method="QLTB", renls2=T,
               control=list(freq=0))
> conf.boot.nl2 <-  bootstrap.nls2(orobranche.nl2,
               method="wild.2",
               n.loops=500)
> delnls2()
```

We calculate the 2.5% and 97.5% quantiles of the $\widehat{T}^{\star,b}$, $b = 1, \ldots 500$, using the function **quantile** of S-Plus, and we display the values of $\widehat{\tau}$, $\widehat{S}$, $b_{0.025}$, $b_{0.975}$, and $\widehat{I}_B$:

```
> tauStar <- conf.boot.nl2$pStar[,5]
> StauStar <- sqrt(conf.boot.nl2$var.pStar[,5])
> qu <- quantile((tauStar-tau)/StauStar,c(0.025,0.975))
> cat("Estimated value of tau:", tau,"\n")
> cat("Estimated value of S:", Stau,"\n")
> cat("b_(0.025):", qu[1],"\n" )
> cat("b_(0.975):", qu[2],"\n" )
> cat("Estimated value of Ib:",
     tau + qu[1]*Stau,
     tau + qu[2]*Stau,"\n")
```

Modeling the Variance Function as in Equation (6.28)

The model is described in a file called **orobranche.m4**:

```
% file orobranche.m4
% logistic regression model
% overdispersion :  beta-binomial variance
resp y;
varind sp,ex,n;
aux eta,p,tau;
var v;
parresp a,b,c,d;
parvar t00, t01, t10, t11;
subroutine;
```

```
begin
eta=a + b*sp + c*ex + d*sp*ex;
p=exp(eta)/(1+exp(eta));
y = n*p;
tau=if ((sp==0)and(ex==0)) then t00 else
    if ((sp==0)and(ex==1)) then t01 else
    if ((sp==1 )and(ex==0)) then t10 else
      t11
fi fi fi;
v = n*(1-p)*p*(1+tau*(n-1));
end
```

Then we call **nls2** as in the preceding example:

```
> ctx <- list( theta.start=orobranche.nl11$theta,
               beta.start=rep(0,4),
               sigma2.type="KNOWN", sigma2=1)
> orobranche.nl4 <- nls2(orobranche, "orobranche.m4",
                         ctx, method="QLTB")
> cat( "Result of the estimation process:\n ")
> print(summary(orobranche.nl4))
```

Modeling the Variance Function as in Equation (6.29)

The model is described in a file called **orobranche.m5**:

```
% file orobranche.m5
% logistic linear regression model
% overdispersion : Gaussian random effect on eta
resp y;
varind sp,ex,n;
aux eta,p;
var v;
parresp a,b,c,d;
parvar tau;
subroutine;
begin
eta=a + b*sp + c*ex + d*sp*ex;
p=exp(eta)/(1+exp(eta));
y = n*p;
v = n*(1-p)*p*(1+(n-1)*tau*p*(1-p));
end
```

Then we call **nls2** as in the preceding example:

```
> ctx <- list( theta.start=orobranche.nl11$theta,
               beta.start=0,
               sigma2.type="KNOWN", sigma2=1)
> orobranche.nl5 <- nls2(orobranche, "orobranche.m5",
                         ctx, method="QLTB")
> cat( "Result of the estimation process:\n ")
> print(summary(orobranche.nl5))
```

7

Multinomial and Poisson Nonlinear Models

In this chapter, we consider two additional statistical models that are very useful for analyzing data sets in agronomy, medicine, and social sciences: The multinomial model and the Poisson model.

The binomial model considered in the preceding chapter deals with response variables with two categories: The occurrence or nonoccurrence of an event is observed. The multinomial model considers multicategory response variables. This topic is discussed in the first part of this chapter. Our objective is not to provide a complete course on the multinomial model (see McCullagh and Nelder [MN89] and Aitkin et al. [AAFH89] for an introduction to this topic). We begin with two examples of multicategory response data and describe the modeling of the probability functions and the quasi-likelihood method for estimating the parameters. Then we demonstrate how to estimate the parameters, calculate confidence intervals, and perform tests, taking full advantage of the nls2's facilities: The relationships between the probability functions and the independent variables do not need to be log-linear; the statistical inference for any parameter function is carried out easily using the same nls2 functions as for the nonlinear regression model.

The second part of the chapter is concerned with count data. We describe how the data from the cortisol assay example presented in Chapter 1 can be fitted using a Poisson nonlinear model. We show how we can easily adapt for overdispersed data using nls2.

7.1 Multinomial Model

We illustrate the use of the multinomial model with two examples that have already been analyzed in the literature. The first example, concerning the study of pneumoconiosis among coal miners, has been analyzed by McCullagh and Nelder [MN89, page 178] and by Aitkin et al. [MAH89, page 225] and the second one, concerning a cheese tasting experiment by McCullagh and

Nelder [MN89, page 175]. We refer to these books for a detailed treatment of these data sets.

7.1.1 Pneumoconiosis among Coal Miners: An Example of Multicategory Response Data

The aim of this experiment is to evaluate the degree of severity of pneumoconiosis in coal miners as a function of time spent working at the coal face. The coal miners are classified by radiological examination into one of three categories of pneumoconiosis: N when the radiological examination is normal, M when it reveals a mild pneumoconiosis, and S for a severe pneumoconiosis. The maximum time spent working at the coal face is 60 years. The interval $[0, 60]$ is partitioned into $k = 8$ intervals and for $i = 1, \ldots, k$ the midpoints of these intervals are denoted by x_i. The number of categories, denoted by r, equals 3, and for $l = 1, \ldots, r$, $Y_{i,l}$ is the number of miners classified in the category l whose time spent working equals x_i (the covariate x takes the value x_i if the time spent working belongs to the interval i). The vector $(Y_{i,1}, \ldots, Y_{i,r})$ is distributed as a multinomial variable with parameters $(p_{i,1}, \ldots, p_{i,r})$ where $p_{i,l}$ denotes the probability of a miner being in category l when the time spent working equals x_i. The results are reported in Table 7.1. As with the binomial model, we describe the relationship between the probability of belonging to one of the categories l versus the covariate x with a parametric function: $p_l(x, \theta)$. This example is used to illustrate the modeling and estimation of the probabilities $p_{i,l}$, $l = 1, \ldots, r$, $i = 1, \ldots, k$ based on the multinomial logit model. We will describe how to estimate the parameters and calculate confidence intervals for the probabilities $p_{i,l}$ using nls2.

Table 7.1. Pneumoconiosis among coal miners

Time	Normal	Mild	Severe	Total
5.8	98	0	0	98
15.0	51	2	1	54
21.5	34	6	3	43
27.5	35	5	8	48
33.5	32	10	9	51
39.5	23	7	8	38
46.0	12	6	10	28
51.5	4	2	5	11

7.1.2 A Cheese Tasting Experiment

This data set concerns the effect on taste of various cheese additives. Four additives labeled A, B, C, and D are tested by 52 panelists. The nine response categories range from "strong dislike" (category I) to "excellent taste" (category IX). The observation, Y_{il}, is the number of panelists that scored the additive x_i (x takes $k = 4$ values, A, B, C, D) in category l, $l = 1, \ldots, r$, with $r = 9$. For each i, the vector $(Y_{i1}, \ldots, Y_{ir})$ is distributed as a multinomial variable with parameters $N = 52$ and $(p_{i,1}, \ldots, p_{i,r})$, where $p_{i,l}$ denotes the probability of an additive x_i receiving the score l. The results are reported in Table 7.2. The same 52 panelists being involved in all four tests, the observations $(Y_{i1}, \ldots, Y_{ir})$ are not independent when i varies. Nevertheless this will be ignored in the analysis (see the comments of McCullagh and Nelder [MN89]).

Table 7.2. Cheese tasting

Cheese	Categories								
	I	II	III	IV	V	VI	VII	VIII	IX
A	0	0	1	7	8	8	19	8	1
B	6	9	12	11	7	6	1	0	0
C	1	1	6	8	23	7	5	1	0
D	0	0	0	1	3	7	14	16	11

This example is used to illustrate the modeling of the probabilities $p_{i,l}$, $l = 1, \ldots, r$, $i = 1, \ldots, k$ in the case of ordered categories; the aim of the analysis is to order the cheeses from best to worst.

7.1.3 The Parametric Multinomial Model

The model is the following. The response variable has r categories, and we observe the response of individuals that belong to one, and only one, of these categories. For each value of the variable x_i, $i = 1, \ldots k$, the responses of N_i individuals are considered: For each $l = 1, \ldots, r$, the observation $Y_{i,l}$ is the number of individuals out of N_i that belong to category l. For each $i = 1, \ldots, k$, the vector $(Y_{i1}, \ldots Y_{ir})$ is distributed as a multinomial variable with parameters N_i and $(p_{i,1}, \ldots, p_{i,r})$, where $p_{i,l}$ denotes the probability of being in category l when the covariate x equals x_i. The probabilities $p_{i,l}$, $l = 1, \ldots, r$, satisfy the following constraint:

$$\text{For each } i = 1, \ldots, k, \ \sum_{l=1}^{r} p_{i,l} = 1. \tag{7.1}$$

We first present a general modeling of the probability functions that includes the well-known *multinomial logit model*. Then we will consider the model adapted to the case of ordered response categories, based on cumulative probabilities.

General Modeling of the Probability Function

Instead of modeling the probabilities $p_{i,l}$ for $l = 1, \ldots, r$ satisfying the constraint defined by Equation (7.1), we consider the quantities $p_{i,l}/p_{i,1}$, or as is usually done, their logarithm. The multinomial logit transformation of $p_{i,1}, \ldots, p_{i,r}$ is the set of parameters $\eta_{i,1}, \ldots, \eta_{i,r}$, called *multinomial logits*, defined by $\eta_{i,l} = \log(p_{i,l}/p_{i,1})$. Let $\eta_l(x, \theta)$ be the function that describes the log-ratio of the probability of being in category l to the probability of being in the reference category when the covariate equals x. The probabilities $p_{i,l}$ are thus written:

$$p_{i,l} = p_l(x_i, \theta) = p_{i,1} \exp\left(\eta_l(x_i, \theta)\right),$$

where for each $i = 1, \ldots, k$, $\eta_1(x_i, \theta) = 0$. The constraint defined by Equation (7.1) being equivalent to

$$p_{i,1} \sum_{l=1}^{r} \exp\left(\eta_l(x_i, \beta)\right) = 1,$$

the probability functions are written as follows:

$$p_l(x_i, \theta) = \frac{\exp\left(\eta_l(x_i, \theta)\right)}{1 + \sum_{s=2}^{r} \exp\left(\eta_s(x_i, \theta)\right)} \quad \text{with} \quad \eta_1(x_i, \theta) = 0. \tag{7.2}$$

The probability functions $p_l(x_i, \theta)$ depend on p unknown parameters θ. Usually, it is assumed that the functions η_l are linear in θ. For the miners example, the following modeling is proposed: For $l = 2, 3$,

$$\eta_l(x_i, \theta) = \theta_{0,l} + \theta_{1,l} \log(x_i). \tag{7.3}$$

As we will see in Section 7.1.8, nls2 allows us to estimate the parameters θ for any parametric function η_l. The relation between η_l and x does not need to be linear in the parameters θ.

Ordered Response Categories

The three categories considered in the miners example are naturally ordered: There is no pneumoconiosis, the pneumoconiosis is mild, the pneumoconiosis is severe. This is also clearly the case in the cheese tasting example: The categories are ordered from the worst to the best. In the case of ordered response categories, it may be of interest to model the *cumulative probabilities* in place of the probabilities $p_{i,l}$. Let us define the cumulative probabilities $P_{i,l}$:

$$P_{i,l} = \sum_{s=1}^{l} p_{i,s},$$

$$P_{i,r} = 1.$$

We immediately see that $p_{i,1} = P_{i,1}$ and $p_{i,l} = P_{i,l} - P_{i,l-1}$ for $l = 2, \ldots, r$. For each $l = 1, \ldots, k$, we denote by $P_l(x_i, \theta)$ the probability of an individual belonging to one of the categories among categories 1 to l, when the covariate x equals x_i. For $i = 1, \ldots, k$, the functions $P_l(x_i, \theta)$ satisfy the following set of constraints:

$$\left. \begin{array}{l} P_r(x_i, \theta) = 1, \\ P_l(x_i, \theta) \geq P_{l-1}(x_i, \theta) \end{array} \right\}. \tag{7.4}$$

Then the probability functions $p_l(x, \theta)$ are written as follows:

$$\left. \begin{array}{l} p_1(x, \theta) = P_1(x, \theta), \\ p_l(x, \theta) = P_l(x, \theta) - P_{l-1}(x, \theta), \text{ for } l = 2, \ldots, r \end{array} \right\}. \tag{7.5}$$

The program nls2 allows us to estimate the parameters θ for any parametric function P_l. Nevertheless let us recall some common methods of modeling these cumulative probability functions. The most famous ones are using the logit or cloglog transformation. It is assumed, for example, that:

$$\begin{array}{l} \text{logit}\,(P_l(x, \theta)) = \theta_{0,l} + \theta_1 x \text{ or} \\ \text{cloglog}\,(P_l(x, \theta)) = \theta_{0,l} + \theta_1 x, \end{array} \tag{7.6}$$

with $\theta_{0,1} \leq \cdots \leq \theta_{0,(r-1)}$. These models involve parallel regressions on the logit or cloglog scale. The one defined by Equation (7.6) is called the proportional odds model and is of interest when the aim of the analysis is to estimate the odds ratio (see [McC80] for details).

Another important class of models considers the existence of a latent variable Z. The latent variable Z is an underlying unobserved continuous random variable with expectation μ, variance $\exp(\tau)$, and distribution function denoted by $F((z - \mu)/\exp(\tau))$. Let $z_1 < \cdots < z_{r-1}$ be some fixed values of Z. Then it is assumed that the probability of belonging to the category l equals the probability of Z belonging to the interval $]z_{l-1}, z_l]$, with $z_0 = -\infty$ and $z_r = +\infty$. Therefore:

$$P_l(x, \theta) = F\left(\frac{z_l - \mu(x, \theta)}{\exp(\tau(x, \theta))}\right).$$

If Z has the logistic distribution, then:

$$\text{logit}\,(P_l(x, \theta)) = \frac{z_l - \mu(x, \theta)}{\exp(\tau(x, \theta))}.$$

If $\tau(x, \theta) = 0$ and μ is linear in the parameters θ, for example, $\mu(x, \theta) = \theta_1 x$, then we get the model defined at Equation (7.6), where the parameters $\theta_{0,l}$ play the role of the thresholds z_l. McCullagh and Nelder [MN89] proposed considering the particular form where μ and τ are linear functions of the parameters, for example, $\mu(x, \theta) = \theta_1 x$ and $\tau(x, \theta) = \theta_2 x$.

7.1.4 Estimation in the Multinomial Model

Let us recall that for each $i = 1, \ldots, k$, the vector $(Y_{i,1}, \ldots Y_{i,r})$ is distributed as a multinomial variable with parameters $N_i = \sum_{l=1}^{r} Y_{i,l}$ and $(p_{i,1}, \ldots, p_{i,r})$. The probabilities $p_{i,l}$ are modeled as follows:

$$p_{i,l} = p_l(x_i, \theta) \tag{7.7}$$

and satisfy the constraints

$$\sum_{l=}^{r} p_l(x_i, \theta) = 1. \tag{7.8}$$

Because the distribution of the observation is known, the parameters are estimated by maximizing the likelihood under the constraints (7.8). The deviance function is defined as

$$D(\theta) = -2 \sum_{i=1}^{k} \sum_{l=1}^{r} Y_{i,l} \log \left(\frac{N_i p_l(x_i, \theta)}{Y_{i,l}} \right), \tag{7.9}$$

where θ denotes the vector of parameters to estimate. The minimum deviance estimator of θ under the constraints (7.8) is the maximum likelihood estimator and is defined as follows: $\widehat{\theta}$ satisfies $U_a(\widehat{\theta}) = 0$, where for $a = 1, \ldots, p$

$$U_a(\theta) = \sum_{i=1}^{k} \sum_{l=1}^{r} \frac{Y_{i,l} - N_i p_l(x_i, \theta)}{N_i p_l(x_i, \theta)} N_i \frac{\partial p_l}{\partial \theta_a}(x_i, \theta). \tag{7.10}$$

To calculate the maximum likelihood estimator of θ using nls2, we use the quasi-likelihood method (see Section 7.1.8).

Let us give some details on the estimating equations given by Equation (7.10). For $(Y_1, \ldots, Y_r)$ a random variable distributed as a multinomial with parameters $N = \sum_{l=1}^{r} Y_l$ and $(p_1, \ldots, p_r)$, we set

$$\ell(y_1, \ldots, y_r, N, p_1, \ldots, p_r) = \Pr(Y_1 = y_1, \ldots, Y_r = y_r) = N! \prod_{l=1}^{r} p_l^{y_l}.$$

Let us denote by $\widetilde{Y}$ the vector of observations:

$$\widetilde{Y} = (Y_{1,1}, \ldots, Y_{1,r}, \ldots, Y_{k,1}, \ldots, Y_{k,r}),$$

and by $\widetilde{p}$ the vector of probabilities:

$$\widetilde{p} = (p_{1,1}, \ldots, p_{1,r}, \ldots, p_{k,1}, \ldots, p_{k,r}),$$

where $p_{i,l}$ is the probability of an individual whose covariate equals x_i belonging to the category l. The likelihood function is defined by the following formula:

$$L(\widetilde{Y}, \widetilde{p}) = \prod_{i=1}^{k} \ell(Y_{i,1}, \ldots, Y_{i,r}, N_i, p_{i,1}, \ldots, p_{i,r}).$$

For i varying from 1 to k, and for l from 1 to r, let

$$\pi_{i,l} = \frac{Y_{i,l}}{N_i}$$

be the empirical frequencies. Then, for a given modeling of the probability function, for example, $p_{i,l} = p_l(x_i, \theta)$, the deviance is defined as

$$D(\theta) = -2 \log \frac{L\left(\widetilde{Y}, \widetilde{p}(\theta)\right)}{L\left(\widetilde{Y}, \widetilde{\pi}\right)},$$

where the components of $\widetilde{p}(\theta)$ and $\widetilde{\pi}$ are, respectively, the quantities $p_l(x_i, \theta)$ and $\pi_{i,l}$. It is easy to verify that we get the formula given in Equation (7.9). The link between the minimum of deviance estimation and the estimating equations given at Equations (7.10) is established by noting that minimizing $D(\theta)$ is equivalent to solving the following equations:

$$\frac{\partial D}{\partial \theta_a}(\theta) = 0, \text{ for } a = 1, \ldots, p.$$

Starting from Equation (7.9), we get the following:

$$\frac{\partial D}{\partial \theta_a}(\theta) = -2 \sum_{i=1}^{k} \sum_{l=1}^{r} \frac{Y_{i,l}}{p_l(x_i, \theta)} \frac{\partial p_l}{\partial \theta_a}(x_i, \theta).$$

Noting that constraint (7.8) implies that the derivatives of $\sum_{l=1}^{r} p_l(x_i, \theta)$ with respect to θ equals 0, we find that:

$$\frac{\partial D}{\partial \theta_a}(\theta) = -2U_a(\theta)$$

where $U_a(\theta)$ is defined at Equation (7.10). Therefore, if $\widehat{\theta}$ minimizes the deviance under the constraint (7.8), then for $a = 1, \ldots, p$, $U_a(\widehat{\theta}) = 0$.

Let us continue these methodological explanations with the link between the multinomial and Poisson likelihoods. First, if we compare Equation (7.10) with Equation (7.19) it appears that the estimating equations in the multinomial model are the same as the estimating equations in the Poisson model if $f(x_i, \theta)$ is replaced by $N_i p_l(x_i, \theta)$, Y_{ij} by $Y_{i,l}$, and if the summation over the indices i and j is replaced by the summation over the indices i and l. Minimizing the deviance in the multinomial model under the constraints $\sum_{l=1}^{r} p_l(x_i, \theta) = 1$ is thus equivalent to minimizing the deviance in the Poisson model. Second, comparing Equation (7.9) with Equation (7.18), it appears that the minimum deviance $D(\widehat{\theta})$ in the multinomial model is the same as the minimum deviance in the Poisson model. These observations are the result of the following statistical argument. Suppose that $Z_1, \ldots, Z_r$ are independent Poisson variables with means $\lambda_1, \ldots, \lambda_r$; then, it can be proved that the joint distribution of $(Z_1, \ldots, Z_r)$ conditional on $\sum_{l=1}^{r} Z_l = N$ is the multinomial distribution:

$$\Pr\left(Z_1 = z_1, \ldots, Z_r = z_r / \sum_{l=1}^{r} z_l = N\right) = \frac{N!}{\left(\sum_{s=1}^{r} \lambda_s\right)^N} \prod_{l=1}^{r} \lambda_l^{z_l}.$$

Setting $Z_l = Y_{i,l}$ and $\lambda_l = N_i p_{i,l}$, the link between the multinomial distribution and the Poisson distribution is clear. People who are familiar with multicategory response data will be used to estimating the probability functions $p_l(x, \theta)$ using a Poisson model. By setting

$$\psi_i = \log(p_{i,1}) = -\log\left[1 + \sum_{s=2}^{r} \exp\left(\eta_s(x_i, \theta)\right)\right],\qquad (7.11)$$

then

$$p_{i,l} = \exp(\psi_i + \eta_l(x_i, \theta)). \qquad (7.12)$$

The probabilities $p_{i,l}$ depend now on $k + p$ parameters: The p parameters θ used in the modeling of the ratios $p_{i,l}/p_{i,1}$ and the k parameters $\psi_1, \ldots, \psi_k$, called *nuisance parameters* because they are not of interest. If the function $\eta_l(x_i, \theta)$ is linear in θ (see, for example, Equation (7.3)), then the Poisson analysis based on a log-linear response can be used for estimating the parameters in the multinomial model. We will come back to the analogy between the Poisson and multinomial analyses later.

7.1.5 Tests and Confidence Intervals

We begin this section with the goodness-of-fit test. It is done exactly as in the binomial model (see Section 6.5, page 167), assuming that for each value of the variable x_i, the total number of individuals N_i is large.

Then we briefly present the calculation of confidence intervals for a function of the parameters, using the Wald test and the likelihood ratio test. We will consider the case where the parameters of interest are the probabilities $p_{i,l}$. For people who are interested in technical backgrounds, we discuss the way the estimated standard error of $\hat{p}_{i,l}$ is calculated, and we point out that the standard outputs of the log-linear Poisson analysis cannot be used.

We do not propose any bootstrap method for calculating confidence intervals in multinomial models.

Goodness-of-Fit Test

Let us consider the multinomial model defined in Equation (7.7) where the dimension of the parameter θ equals p. Assume that for each $i = 1, \ldots, k$ the quantities N_i are large.

Testing goodness of fit consists of testing the model (7.7) against the saturated model defined as follows: For each $i = 1, \ldots, k$, the vector $(Y_{i,1}, \ldots Y_{i,r})$ is distributed as a multinomial variable with parameters $N_i = \sum_{l=1}^{r} Y_{i,l}$ and $(p_{i,1}, \ldots, p_{i,r})$. The $p_{i,l}$s, for $i = 1, \ldots, k$ and $l = 1, \ldots, r - 1$ are the $k(r - 1)$ parameters of the model. The maximum likelihood estimators of the probabilities $p_{i,l}$ are the empirical frequencies $\pi_{i,l} = Y_{i,l}/N_i$, and the likelihood ratio test is the deviance associated with the model (7.7). Therefore the goodness-of-fit test is rejected when $D(\hat{\theta})$ is greater than C, where C is the $1 - \alpha$ quantile of a χ^2 with $k(r - 1) - p$ degrees of freedom.

The likelihood ratio test

The likelihood ratio test for comparing two nested models is done exactly as described for the binomial model, using the deviance statistic (see Section 6.5, page 165). In the same way, we can calculate confidence regions or confidence intervals for the parameters θ.

The Wald Test

The Wald test for comparing two nested models or calculating confidence intervals for a function of the parameters is done exactly as in Section 3.4.1, page 69.

Suppose that we want to calculate a confidence interval for a function of the parameters denoted $\lambda(\theta)$, for example, $\lambda(\theta) = p_1(x_i, \theta)$ for some i. The 95% confidence interval based on the Wald statistic is defined as

$$\widehat{I}_N = \left[\widehat{\lambda} - 1.96\widehat{S}; \widehat{\lambda} + 1.96\widehat{S}\right],$$

where $\widehat{\lambda} = \lambda(\widehat{\theta}) = p_1(x_i, \widehat{\theta})$, and $\widehat{S}$ is an estimate of the standard error of $\widehat{\lambda}$. If we test hypothesis H: $\lambda = \lambda_0$ against the alternative A: $\lambda \neq \lambda_0$, the Wald statistic is defined as

$$\mathcal{S}_W = \frac{(\widehat{\lambda} - \lambda_0)^2}{\widehat{S}^2}.$$

If the parameters are estimated by introducing the nuisance parameters $\psi_1, \ldots, \psi_k$ and using the link between the log-linear Poisson model and the multinomial model, then $\lambda = \exp(\psi_i)$, and the estimated variance of $\widehat{\lambda}$ is approximated by $\exp(2\widehat{\psi_i})\mathrm{Var}(\widehat{\psi_i})$. We will show that we cannot use the standard outputs of the program minimizing the Poisson likelihood for estimating the variance of $\widehat{\psi_i}$.

Let us return to the general case where $\lambda = \lambda(\theta)$. Because the estimated standard error $\widehat{S}$ of $\lambda(\widehat{\theta})$ is a function of the estimated covariance matrix of $\widehat{\theta}$ (see Equation (2.1), page 32), let us see how this covariance matrix is calculated.

The programs solving the estimating equations defined in Equation (7.10) calculate the estimated covariance matrix of $\widehat{\theta}$ assuming that the variables $Y_{i,l}, l = 1, \ldots, r, i = 1,, \ldots, k$ are independent with expectation and variance equal to $N_i p_l(x_i, \theta)$. Namely, it is assumed that the covariance matrix of $Y_{i,l}, l = 1, \ldots, r$ equals the diagonal matrix W_i^P whose components on the diagonal equal $N_i p_l(x_i, \theta)$, for $l = 1, \ldots, r$.

In the case of multinomial observations, this is not true: The $Y_{i,l}, l = 1, \ldots, r$ are not independent, and it is well known that the covariance matrix of $Y_{i,l}, l = 1, \ldots, r$ is the matrix W_i^M whose components (l, s) are equal to $\mathrm{Cov}(Y_{i,l}, Y_{i,s})$, for $l, s = 1, \ldots, k$ where

$$\mathrm{Var}(Y_{i,l}) = N_i p_l(x_i, \theta)(1 - p_l(x_i, \theta)),$$
$$\mathrm{Cov}(Y_{i,l}, Y_{i,s}) = -N_i p_l(x_i, \theta) p_s(x_i, \theta).$$

Nevertheless, it can be shown that:

1. the asymptotic covariance matrix of $\widehat{\theta}$ is the same as the matrix we would have obtained using W_i^P in place of W_i^M, and

2. if the modeling of the probability functions depends on nuisance parameters (see Equations (7.11) and (7.12)), then the result is true for $\widehat{\theta}$ but not for $\widehat{\psi}$.

As a consequence, if the function λ depends on ψ (for example, $\lambda = p_{i,1} = \exp(\psi_i)$) the standard outputs of the program used for estimating the parameters in the Poisson model cannot be used to calculate the estimated standard error $\widehat{S}$. It is thus of interest to estimate the parameters θ using nls2: This program does not require introducing nuisance parameters in the estimation process and proposes an easy-to-use function (see the function confidence.nls2, Section 7.1.8) for calculating confidence intervals for any parameter function.

7.1.6 Pneumoconiosis among Coal Miners: The Multinomial Logit Model

Model The observations $(Y_{i,1}, \ldots, Y_{i,r})$, $i = 1, \ldots, k$ are multinomial variables with parameters N_i and

$$p_l(x_i, \theta) = \frac{\exp\left(\eta_l(x_i, \theta)\right)}{1 + \sum_{s=2}^r \eta_s(x_i, \theta)}. \tag{7.13}$$

The model is the multinomial logit model, where the relationship between η_l and $\log(x)$ is linear in θ:

$$\left.\begin{array}{l} \eta_1(x_i, \theta) = 0, \\ \eta_l(x_i, \theta) = \theta_{0,l} + \theta_{1,l} \log(x_i). \text{ for } l = 2, 3 \end{array}\right\}. \tag{7.14}$$

Method The parameters are estimated by minimizing the deviance $D(\theta)$ (see Equation (7.9)).

Results

Parameters β	Estimated Values	Standard Error
$\theta_{0,2}$	-8.93	1.58
$\theta_{1,2}$	2.16	0.46
$\theta_{0,3}$	-11.9	2.00
$\theta_{1,3}$	3.07	0.56

Goodness-of-Fit Test and Graphics for Diagnostic The minimum deviance $D(\widehat{\theta})$ equals 5.35. Using the results of Section 7.1.5, we test the hypothesis that the probability function is the function defined by Equations (7.13) and (7.14) with four parameters against the alternative that $p_l(x_i, \theta) = p_{i,l}$ with $k(r-1) = 16$ parameters. Because the 0.95 quantile of a χ^2 with 12 degrees of freedom is equal to 21, the goodness-of-fit test is not rejected.

Let us now examine the observations together with the result of the estimation. We calculate the standardized residuals defined as in the binomial model:

$$\widehat{e}_{i,l} = \frac{Y_{i,l} - N_i \widehat{p}_{i,l}}{\sqrt{N_i \widehat{p}_{i,l}(1 - \widehat{p}_{i,l})}}, \tag{7.15}$$

where $\widehat{p}_{i,l} = p_l(x_i, \widehat{\theta})$. The plot of residuals is shown in Figure 7.1. This figure shows that the probability of having pneumoconiosis is overestimated when the time spent working is less than 20 years. It does not show any other particular model specification.

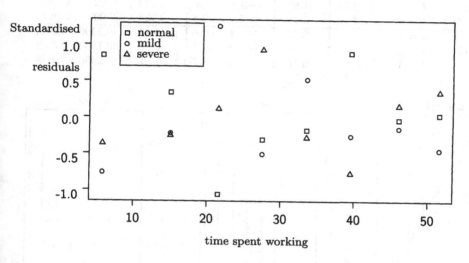

Figure 7.1. Pneumoconiosis among coal miners example: Multinomial logit model

Figure 7.2 represents on the same graph the empirical frequencies, the fitted probabilities, and their confidence intervals.

Calculation of Confidence Intervals for the Probabilities $p_{i,l}$ Because the probabilities are positive quantities, it is generally preferable to calculating confidence intervals for their logarithm. We first calculate $\widehat{I}_{\mathcal{N}}(i, l)$, the confidence interval for $\log(p_{i,l})$. Then we take the exponential of each bound of this interval.

Result

We denote by $\widehat{S}(i, l)$ the estimated standard error of $\log(p_{i,l})$. The 95% confidence interval for $p_l(x_i, \theta)$ is denoted by $\exp\left(\widehat{I}_{\mathcal{N}}(i, l)\right)$. To be brief: We present the numerical results for only two values of the time spent working in Table 7.3. All the results are presented in Figure 7.2. It appears that the variability of the estimated probabilities is very large.

Table 7.3. Pneumoconiosis among coal miners example: Confidence intervals for $p_{i,l}$ for x_i equals 15 and 46

Time	Category	$\log(\widehat{p}_{i,l})$	$\widehat{S}(i,l)$	$\widehat{I}_{\mathcal{N}}(i,l)$	$\widehat{p}_{i,l}$	$\exp\left(\widehat{I}_{\mathcal{N}}(i,l)\right)$
	$l = 1$	-0.07	0.02	$[-0.11 \; ; -0.03]$	0.93	$[0.9000 \; ; 0.970]$
15	$l = 2$	-3.10	0.36	$[-3.8 \; ; -2.4 \,]$	0.043	$[0.0210 \; ; 0.088]$
	$l = 3$	-3.70	0.48	$[-4.7 \; ; -2.8 \,]$	0.024	$[0.0093 \; ; 0.061]$
	$l = 1$	-0.84	0.12	$[-1.1 \; ; -0.6 \,]$	0.43	$[0.3400 \; ; 0.540]$
46	$l = 2$	-1.50	0.19	$[-1.9 \; ; -1.1 \,]$	0.23	$[0.1600 \; ; 0.330]$
	$l = 3$	1.10	0.16	$[-1.4 \; ; -0.77]$	0.34	$[0.2500 \; ; 0.460]$

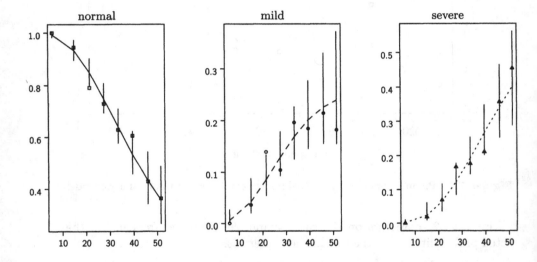

Figure 7.2. Pneumoconiosis among coal miners example: Model based on cumulative probabilities; empirical frequencies versus time spent working, fitted probabilities, and estimated confidence intervals at level 95%

7.1.7 Cheese Tasting Example: Model Based on Cumulative Probabilities

The observations $(Y_{i,1}, \dots, Y_{i,r})$, $i = 1, \dots, k$ are multinomial variables with parameters $N = 52$ and $p_l(x_i, \theta)$ defined in Equation (7.5). The function $P_l(x, \theta)$ is the probability for an additive x having a score smaller than l. We consider the model based on a latent variable with a logistic distribution with expectation $\theta_{1,i}$ and variance 1: For $i = 1, \dots, 4$,

$$\text{logit}(P_l(x_i, \theta)) = \theta_{0,l} - \theta_{1,i}, \text{ for } l = 1, \dots, 8,$$
$$P_9(x, \theta) = 1.$$

The parameters θ must satisfy $\theta_{0,l} \leq \theta_{0,l+1}$ for $l = 1, \ldots, 7$. This constraint can be taken into account in the estimation process by changing the parameterization: For example, by setting, $\theta_{0,l} = \theta_{0,1} + \sum_{s=2}^{l} \exp(\theta_{2,l})$, for $l = 2, \ldots, 8$. The parameters $\theta_{0,1}, \theta_{2,2}, \ldots, \theta_{2,8}$ are then estimated in place of $\theta_{0,1}, \ldots, \theta_{0,8}$. Moreover, the parameters θ are defined up to a constant, and we will assume that $\sum_{i=1}^{4} \theta_{1,i} = 0$, such that the model is identifiable.

Method The parameters are estimated by minimizing the deviance $D(\theta)$ (see Equation (7.9)) under the constraints $P_9(x, \theta) = 1$ and $\sum_{i=1}^{4} \theta_{1,i} = 0$.

Result The results are given in Table 7.4. The estimated value of the parameter $\theta_{1,4}$ is calculated from the estimations of $(\theta_{1,1}, \theta_{1,2}, \theta_{1,3})$. We get $\widehat{\theta}_{1,4} = -2.47$, and the estimated standard error equals 0.27.

Table 7.4. Cheese tasting. Estimated values of the parameters and their standard errors

Parameters θ	Estimated Values	Standard Error
$\theta_{0,1}$	−4.6	0.426
$\theta_{2,2}$	0.054	0.30
$\theta_{2,3}$	0.095	0.21
$\theta_{2,4}$	0.066	0.18
$\theta_{2,5}$	0.29	0.15
$\theta_{2,6}$	−0.049	0.18
$\theta_{2,7}$	0.41	0.15
$\theta_{2,8}$	0.44	0.18
$\theta_{1,1}$	−0.86	0.23
$\theta_{1,2}$	2.49	0.27
$\theta_{1,3}$	0.85	0.23

Goodness-of-Fit Test and Graphics for Diagnostic Using the results of Section 7.1.5, we test goodness of fit by comparing the preceding model with 11 parameters to the saturated model with 32 parameters, where the variables $(Y_{i,1}, \ldots, Y_{i,r})$, $i = 1, \ldots, k$ are multinomial variables with parameters N and p_{il}. The minimum deviance $D(\widehat{\theta}) = 20.3$ has to be compared to 32.7, the 0.95 quantile of a χ^2 with 21 degrees of freedom. The goodness-of-fit test is not rejected.

Because in this example we are interested in classifying the additives A, B, C, and D, the functions of interest are the cumulative probabilities P_l rather than the probability functions p_l. It is thus appropriate to represent the cumulative observations together with the fitted cumulative probabilities in order to appreciate the quality of the fit. The cumulative observations and the cumulative fitted responses are defined here:

$$Z_{i,l} = \sum_{s=1}^{l} Y_{i,s},$$
$$\widehat{P}_{i,l} = P_l(x_i, \widehat{\theta}) \text{ for } l = 1, \dots, r-1,$$
$$\widehat{P}_{i,r} = 1.$$

The *cumulative residuals* are then defined as follows:

$$\widehat{c}_{i,l} = \frac{Z_{i,l} - N_i \widehat{P}_{i,l}}{N_i \widehat{P}_{i,l}(1 - \widehat{P}_{i,l})} \text{ for } l = 1, \dots, r-1. \qquad (7.16)$$

Note that the $\widehat{c}_{i,r}$s equal 0, because $Z_{i,r} = N_i$. The plots of cumulative residuals are shown in Figure 7.3. The cumulative observations and fitted cumulative responses versus l are shown in Figure 7.4. For each $l = 1, \dots, r-1$ and each $i = 1, \dots, k$, we calculated a confidence interval for the fitted cumulative probabilities.

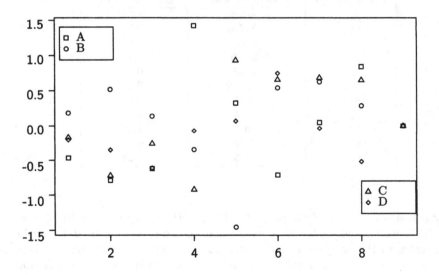

Figure 7.3. Cheese tasting example: Cumulative residuals, $\widehat{c}_{i,l}$, versus the score l.

Confidence Interval for $P_l(x_i, \widehat{\theta})$ *Based on the Wald Test* Because the functions P_l are linear in the parameters through a logit transformation, it is natural to calculate $\widehat{I}_N(i, l)$, the confidence interval for $L_l(x_i, \theta) = \text{logit}(P_l(x_i, \theta))$, and then to transform each bound with the inverse logit function:

$$\text{logit}^{-1}(\eta) = \frac{\exp(\eta)}{1 + \exp(\eta)}.$$

The confidence interval for $P_l(x_i, \widehat{\theta})$ is denoted $\widehat{I}_{\mathcal{N}}(P_{i,l})$.

Results We denote by $\widehat{S}(i, l)$ the estimated standard error of $\mathrm{logit}(P_l(x_i, \widehat{\theta}))$. To be brief, we present the numerical results for $l = 5$ only, the whole analysis being represented in Figure 7.4. Even if the variability in the estimated cumulative probabilities is large, it appears that the cheese additives can be ordered from best to worst as follows: D, A, C, B. Because the confidence intervals for the cumulative probabilities do not overlap, we can conclude that the differences between the additives are significant.

Additive i	$L_5(x_i, \widehat{\theta})$	$\widehat{S}(i, 5)$	$\widehat{I}_{\mathcal{N}}(i, 5)$	$P_5(x_i, \widehat{\theta})$	$\widehat{I}_{\mathcal{N}}(P_{i,5})$
A	-0.9	0.27	$[-1.4; -0.4]$	0.29	$[0.19; 0.41]$
B	2.4	0.34	$[1.8; 3.1]$	0.92	$[0.86; 0.96]$
C	0.8	0.27	$[0.3; 1.3]$	0.69	$[0.57; 0.79]$
D	-2.5	0.34	$[-3.2; -1.8]$	0.074	$[0.039; 0.14]$

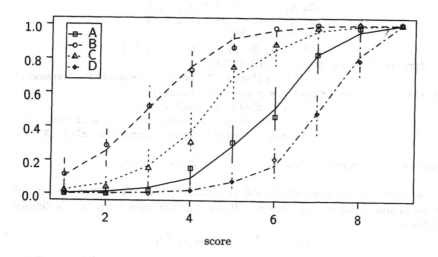

Figure 7.4. Cheese tasting example: Cumulative empirical frequencies and fitted probabilities versus the score l

7.1.8 Using nls2

If the relationships between the probability functions and the independent variables are assumed to be log-linear then the functions **glm** and **multinom** in S-Plus can be used. The program **nls2** allows us to estimate the parameters for any modeling of the probability functions $p_l(x_i, \theta)$ and to calculate confidence intervals or perform tests for any function of the parameters.

This section reproduces the commands and files used in the preceding sections to analyze the examples using **nls2**. For each of them, first we create the *data frame* to store the experimental data, and then we estimate the parameters using the quasi-likelihood method.

Pneumoconiosis among Coal Miners

Creating the Data

The experimental data (see Table 7.1, page 200) are stored in a **matrix** called **miners.data**. Before using **nls2**, this **matrix** is transformed in a **data.frame** called **miners** with three independent variables, **t** contains the x_is replicated r times, **n** is the N_is replicated $r = 3$ times, and **cat** is the categories l, each value being replicated $k = 8$ times, and the variable of observed responses **y** that contains the $Y_{i,l}$s.

```
> miners.data <- t(matrix(c(5.8,98, 0, 0,15.0,51, 2, 1
              ,21.5,34, 6, 3,27.5,35, 5, 8
              ,33.5,32,10, 9,39.5,23, 7, 8
              ,46.0,12, 6,10
              ,51.5, 4, 2, 5), nrow=4,ncol=8))
> dimnames(miners.data) <- list(NULL,
                    c("period","normal","abnormal","severe"))
> miners <- data.frame( t = rep(miners.data[,1],3),
                    y = c(miners.data[,2:4]),
                    n = rep(apply(miners.data[, 2:4],1,sum),3),
                    cat = rep(1:3,rep(dim(miners.data)[1],3)))
```

Parameter Estimation by Minimizing the Deviance Function

In order to solve the quasi-likelihood Equations (7.10), we have to define the regression and variance functions as follows. The regression function is defined as follows:

$$f(x_i, N_i, l; \theta) = N_i p_l(x_i, \theta),$$

where the probability functions p_l are given by Equation (7.13) and (7.14), page 208. The variance function is defined as $g(x_i, N_i, l; \theta) = f(x_i, N_i, l; \theta)$ and $\sigma^2 = 1$.

We describe the model in a file called **miners.m**.

```
%  file miners.m
%  multinomial logit model
resp y;
varind t, n, cat;
aux p, eta, eta2, eta3;
var v;
parresp a2,b2,a3,b3;
subroutine;
```

```
begin
eta3 = a3 + b3*log(t) ;
eta2 = a2 + b2*log(t) ;
eta  = if (cat==3) then eta3 else
          if (cat==2) then eta2 else
          0
fi fi;
p = exp(eta)/(1+exp(eta2)+exp(eta3)) ;
y = n*p;
v = n*p;
end
```

We call `nls2` using its arguments as follows:

- The argument `method`—because minimizing the deviance $D(\theta)$ is equivalent to solving the quasi-likelihood equations defined by Equations (7.10), we will use `nls2` by setting the argument `method` to the value `"QLT"`.
- The argument `stat.ctx`—we have to use the components `sigma2.type` and `sigma2` of the argument `stat.ctx` that describes the statistical context of the analysis. By setting `sigma2.type` to the value `"KNOWN"` and `sigma2` to the value 1, we specify that σ^2 is known and equal to 1. Therefore σ^2 will not be estimated by the residual variance but will stay fixed to the value 1 throughout the estimation process.

  Moreover, the calculations of the maximum likelihood, the minimum deviance, and the standardized residuals will be done only if the component `family` is set to the value `"multinomial"` and if the component `nameN` contains the name of the variable N in the *data frame* containing the data:

```
> ctx <- list(theta.start=rep(0,4),
              sigma2.type="KNOWN", sigma2=1,
              family="multinomial", nameN="n")
> miners.nl1 <- nls2(miners, "miners.m", stat.ctx=ctx, method="QLT")
```

Then we display the result of the estimation process (see page 208):

```
> cat( "Result of the estimation process:\n ")
> print(summary(miners.nl1))
```

Goodness-of-Fit Test

The minimum deviance is given in the output argument `miners.nl1$deviance`. We display its value and the 0.95 quantile of a χ^2 with 12 degrees of freedom:

```
> cat( "Minimum deviance:", miners.nl1$deviance,
       "X2(0.95,12)", qchisq(0.95,12), "\n\n" )
```

Plots of the Residuals

The standardized residuals defined in Equation (7.15), page 208, are given in the output argument `miners.nl1$s.residuals`. The graphic of residuals is done using the graphical function `plres` (see Figure 7.1).

Confidence Intervals for the Probabilities $p_l(x_i, \theta)$

We describe the functions $\log(p_l(x_i, \theta))$ in a file called `miners.log.proba.m`.
Because the probability functions depend on the independent variables, we
use the key word `varpsi`:

```
%    file miners.log.proba.m
%    probabilities
psi logproba;
varpsi t,   cat;
ppsi a2,b2,a3,b3;
aux eta3, eta2, eta;
subroutine;
begin
eta3 = a3 + b3*log(t) ;
eta2 = a2 + b2*log(t) ;
eta  = if (cat==3) then eta3 else
       if (cat==2) then eta2 else
       0
fi fi;
logproba = eta - log(1+exp(eta2)+exp(eta3)) ;
end
```

To calculate a confidence interval for $\log(p_l(x_i, \theta))$, we apply the `confidence`
function. Then we display the results of interest (see Table 7.3, page 210):

```
> loadnls2(psi="")
> lp.conf <- confidence(miners.nl1,
                        file="mineurs.log.proba.m",
                        varpsi=as.matrix(miners[,c(1,4)]))
> IN <- lp.conf$normal.conf.int
> exp.IN <- exp(IN)
> result <- cbind(lp.conf$psi, lp.conf$std.error, IN,
>                 exp(lp.conf$psi), exp.IN)
> dimnames(result) <- list(NULL,c("log.p","Std.log.p","lower.IN",
                      "upper.IN","p","lower.exp.IN","upper.exp.IN"))
> cat("Confidence intervals:","\n")
> print(signif(result,digits=3))
```

The plots of empirical frequencies, fitted probabilities, and confidence intervals versus the time spent working are drawn by the graphical functions of
S-Plus (see Figure 7.2):

```
> p <- miners.nl1$response/miners$n
> freq <- miners.data[,2:4]/apply(miners.data[,2:4],1,sum)
> title <- c("normal", "mild", "severe")
> time <- miners.data[,1]
> par(mfrow=c(1,3))
> for (l in 1:3) {
>   plot(range(time),
```

```
>        range(c(freq[,1],p[(1-1)*8+(1:8)],exp.IN[(1-1)*8+(1:8),])),
>        type="n", xlab="", ylab="")
> points(time, freq[,1], pch=rep(14+1,8))
> lines( time,  p[(1-1)*8+(1:8)], lty=1)
> title(main=title[1])
> segments(time, exp.IN[(1-1)*8+(1:8),1],
>          time, exp.IN[(1-1)*8+(1:8),2])
> }
```

Cheese Tasting

Creating the Data

The experimental data (see Table 7.2, page 201) are stored in a `matrix` called `cheese.data`. Before using `nls2`, this `matrix` is transformed in a `data.frame` called `cheese` with two independent variables and the variable of observed responses +y that contains the $Y_{i,l}$s. The two independent variables are `ch`, which contains the x_is replicated $r = 9$ times, and `cat`, which contains the categories l, each value being replicated $k = 4$ times:

```
> cheese.data <- t(matrix(c(0,0,1,7,8,8,19,8,1,
                            6,9,12,11,7,6,1,0,0,
                            1,1,6,8,23,7,5,1,0,
                            0,0,0,1,3,7,14,16,11),nrow=9,ncol=4))
> cheese <- data.frame(ch=rep(1:4,9),
                       y=c(cheese.data[,1:9]),
                       cat=rep(1:9,rep(4,9)))
```

Parameter Estimation by Minimizing the Deviance Function

In order to solve the quasi-likelihood Equations (7.10), we have to define the regression and variance functions as described for the miners in the example given page 214. We describe the model in a file called `cheese.m`:

```
%   file cheese.m
%   Cumulative probabilities  multinomial model
resp y;
varind  cat, ch;
aux p,beta,pc1,pc2,pc3,pc4,pc5,pc6,pc7,pc8,pc9,
    b2,b3,b4,b5,b6,b7,b8;
var v;
parresp teta1,teta2,teta3,teta4,teta5,teta6,teta7,
        teta8,beta1,beta2,beta3;
subroutine;
begin
beta = if (ch==1) then beta1 else
       if (ch==2) then beta2 else
       if (ch==3) then beta3 else
```

```
            -beta1-beta2-beta3
            fi fi fi;
b2  = teta1 + exp(teta2);
b3  = b2 + exp(teta3);
b4  = b3 + exp(teta4);
b5  = b4 + exp(teta5);
b6  = b5 + exp(teta6);
b7  = b6 + exp(teta7);
b8  = b7 + exp(teta8);
pc1 = exp(teta1+beta)/(1+exp(teta1+beta)) ;
pc2 = exp(b2+beta)/(1+exp(b2+beta)) ;
pc3 = exp(b3+beta)/(1+exp(b3+beta)) ;
pc4 = exp(b4+beta)/(1+exp(b4+beta)) ;
pc5 = exp(b5+beta)/(1+exp(b5+beta)) ;
pc6 = exp(b6+beta)/(1+exp(b6+beta)) ;
pc7 = exp(b7+beta)/(1+exp(b7+beta)) ;
pc8 = exp(b8+beta)/(1+exp(b8+beta)) ;
pc9 = 1;
p   = if (cat==2) then pc2-pc1 else
      if (cat==3) then pc3-pc2 else
      if (cat==4) then pc4-pc3 else
      if (cat==5) then pc5-pc4 else
      if (cat==6) then pc6-pc5 else
      if (cat==7) then pc7-pc6 else
      if (cat==8) then pc8-pc7 else
      if (cat==9) then pc9-pc8 else
      pc1
fi fi fi fi fi fi fi fi;
y = 52*p;
v = 52*p;
end
```

We call nls2 using its arguments as described page 215 for the miners example:

- The argument method is set to the value "QLT".
- The components sigma2.type and sigma2 of the argument stat.ctx are set to the values "KNOWN" and 1, respectively; the components family is set to the value "multinomial"; and nameN is set to the value "n":

```
> ctx <- list(theta.start=c(-8,rep(0,7),rep(0,3)),
            sigma2.type="KNOWN", sigma2=1,
            family="multinomial", nameN="n")
> cheese.nl1 <- nls2(cheese, "cheese.m", stat.ctx=ctx, method="QLT")
```

Then we display the result of the estimation process (see Table 7.4, page 211):

```
> cat( "Result of the estimation process:\n ")
> print(summary(cheese.nl1))
```

Calculation of a confidence interval for $\theta_{1,4}$

The confidence interval based on the Wald test is calculated using the function
confidence. We describe the function $\theta_{1,4} = \lambda(\theta) = -\theta_{1,1} - \theta_{1,2} - \theta_{1,3}$ in a
file called **cheese.teta14.m**:

```
%    file cheese.teta14.m
psi t4;
ppsi beta1,beta2,beta3;
subroutine;
begin
t4 = -beta1-beta2-beta3;
end
```

We apply the **confidence** function and display the estimated value of θ_{14},
its standard error, and confidence interval:

```
> loadnls2(psi="")
> teta14.conf <- confidence(cheese.nl1,
                            file="cheese.teta14.m")
> result <- c(teta14.conf$psi, teta14.conf$std.error,
              teta14.conf$normal.conf.int)
> names(result) <- c("teta14", "std.teta14", "lower.IN", "upper.IN")
> cat("Confidence interval:","\n")
> print(result)
```

Goodness-of-Fit Test

The minimum deviance is given in the output argument **cheese.nl1$deviance**.
We display its value and the 0.95 quantile of a χ^2 with 21 degrees of freedom:

```
> cat( "Minimum deviance:", cheese.nl1$deviance,
       "X2(0.95,21)", qchisq(0.95,21), "\n\n" )
```

Plot of Cumulative Residuals

The standardized residuals defined in Equation (7.16), page 212, are calculated
and plotted using the S-Plus functions (see Figure 7.3):

```
> r <- length(unique(cheese$cat))
> k <- length(unique(cheese$ch))
> n <- rep(52,length(cheese$ch))
> p <- cheese.nl6$response/n
> P <- rep(1,length(p))
> PI <- P
> P[cheese$cat==1] <- p[cheese$cat==1]
> PI[cheese$cat==1] <- cheese$y[cheese$cat==1]/n[cheese$cat==1]
> for (l in (2:r)) {
>    P[cheese$cat==l] <- P[cheese$cat==(l-1)] + p[cheese$cat==l]
>    PI[cheese$cat==l] <- PI[cheese$cat==(l-1)] +
```

```
>                                cheese$y[cheese$cat==1]/n[cheese$cat==1]
> }
> RES <- (n*PI-n*P)/sqrt(n*P*(1-P))
> RES[cheese$cat==r] <- 0
> plot(c(1,r), range(RES), type="n", xlab="score",
        ylab="cumulative standardised residuals",las=1)
> matpoints(1:r, t(matrix(RES,nrow=k)), pch=15:18)
> title <- c("A","B","C","D")
> legend(x=0.8, y=1.4, legend=title, pch=15:18, col=1:4)
```

Confidence Intervals for the Cumulative Probabilities $P_l(x_i, \theta)$

We describe the functions $\text{logit}(P_l(x_i, \theta))$ in a file called **cheese.logit.Proba.m**.
Because the probability functions depend on the independent variables, we use
the key word **varpsi**:

```
%    file cheese.logit.Proba.m
%    cumulative probabilities
psi lProba;
varpsi  cat, ch;
ppsi teta1,teta2,teta3,teta4,teta5,teta6,teta7,
     teta8,beta1,beta2,beta3;
aux  beta,  b2, b3, b4, b5, b6, b7, b8;
subroutine;
begin
beta = if (ind==1) then beta1 else
        if (ind==2) then beta2 else
        if (ind==3) then beta3 else
        - beta1- beta2-beta3
        fi fi fi;
b2  = teta1 + exp(teta2);
b3  = b2 + exp(teta3);
b4  = b3 + exp(teta4);
b5  = b4 + exp(teta5);
b6  = b5 + exp(teta6);
b7  = b6 + exp(teta7);
b8  = b7 + exp(teta8);
lProba = if (cat==2) then b2+beta else
         if (cat==3) then b3+beta else
       if (cat==4) then b4+beta else
       if (cat==5) then b5+beta else
       if (cat==6) then b6+beta else
       if (cat==7) then b7+beta else
       if (cat==8) then b8+beta else
       if (cat==9) then 1 else
       teta1+beta
fi fi fi fi fi fi fi fi;
end
```

To calculate a confidence interval for $\text{logit}(P_l(x_i, \theta))$, we apply the `confidence` function. Then we display the results of interest (see page 213):

```
> loadnls2(psi="")
> 1P.conf <- confidence( cheese.nl1,
            file="cheese.logit.Proba.m",
            varpsi=as.matrix(don_as.matrix(cheese[,c(1,3)])))
> conf.int <- 1P.conf$normal.conf.int
> IN <- exp(conf.int)/(1+exp(conf.int))
> result <- cbind(1P.conf$psi, 1P.conf$std.error,
            1P.conf$normal.conf.int,
            exp(1P.conf$psi)/(1+exp(1P.conf$psi)), IN)
> dimnames(result) <- list(NULL, c("logit.P", "std.logit.P",
            "lower.logit.IN", "upper.logit.IN",
            "P", "lower.1.IN", "upper.1.IN" ))
> cat("Confidence intervals:","\n")
> print(signif(result,digits=3))
```

The plots of cumulative empirical frequencies, fitted probabilities, and confidence intervals versus the score are drawn by the graphical functions of S-Plus (see Figure 7.4):

```
> plot(c(1,r), range(c(PI,P,IN)), type="n",
      xlab="score", ylab="", las=1)
> matpoints(1:r, t(matrix(PI,nrow=4)), pch=15:18)
> matlines(1:r, t(matrix(P,nrow=4)), lty=1:4)
> legend(x=1, y=1, legend=title, lty=1:4, pch=15:18, col=1:4)
> for (l in 1:k) {
>     segments(x0=1:r, y0=IN[cheese$ch==1,1],
>              x1=1:r, y1=IN[cheese$ch==1,2],
>              lty=1)
> }
```

7.2 Poisson Model

In Example 1.1.2, we estimated the calibration curve of a radioimmunological assay of cortisol where, for known dilutions of a purified hormone, the responses are measured in terms of radiation counts per minute (c.p.m.). In Chapter 4, we concluded that a satisfying nonlinear regression model to analyze the cortisol assay data was based on an asymmetric sigmoidally shaped regression function

$$f(x, \theta) = \theta_1 + \frac{\theta_2 - \theta_1}{(1 + \exp(\theta_3 + \theta_4 x))^{\theta_5}} \tag{7.17}$$

with heteroscedastic variances $\text{Var}(\varepsilon_{ij}) = \sigma^2 f^2(x_i, \theta)$. The parameters were estimated by the method of maximum likelihood.

Because the observations are counts that can safely be assumed to be distributed as Poisson variables, we reanalyze the data using the Poisson model. However, as mentioned earlier, departures from the idealized Poisson model are to be suspected: Table 1.3 displays clear evidence that the responses are more variable than the simple Poisson model would suggest. This was accounted for in Chapter 4 by taking an estimate of the variance function proportional to the square of the mean function. We will show how to treat the problem of overdispersion in a Poisson model using the quasi-likelihood method available in **nls2**.

7.2.1 The Parametric Poisson Model

The model is the following: For each value of the covariable x_i and for each replicate $j = 1, \ldots, n_i$, the responses Y_{ij} are independent Poisson variables with mean $f(x_i, \theta)$. The mean function is a nonlinear function of p unknown parameters θ. This modeling extends the *log-linear models* where the logarithm of the mean is a linear function of θ.

In some situations, the dispersion of the data is greater than that predicted by the Poisson model, i.e., $\text{Var}(Y) > \text{E}(Y)$. This heterogeneity has to be taken into account in the modeling of the variance function. For example, if the mean of the observed count, namely $\mu(x, \theta) = \text{E}(Y)$, is regarded as a gamma random variable with expectation $f(x, \theta)$ and variance $f^2(x, \theta)$, then Y is distributed as a negative binomial distribution and the variance function is quadratic instead of linear: $\text{Var}(Y) = f(x, \theta) + f^2(x, \theta)/\tau$. For more details on the modeling of overdispersion of count data, see McCullagh and Nelder [MN89, page 198]. Following the modeling of the variance proposed in Chapter 3, we will assume that the variance varies as a power of the mean $\text{Var}(Y) = \sigma^2 f^\tau(x, \theta)$ and estimate τ.

7.2.2 Estimation in the Poisson Model

The deviance function is defined as follows:

$$D(\theta) = -2 \sum_{i=1}^{k} \sum_{j=1}^{n_i} Y_{ij} \log \left(\frac{f(x_i, \theta)}{Y_{ij}} \right) + Y_{ij} - f(x_i, \theta). \qquad (7.18)$$

The minimum deviance estimator of θ is the maximum likelihood estimator and is defined as follows: $\widehat{\theta}$ satisfies $U_a(\widehat{\theta}) = 0$, where for $a = 1, \ldots, p$

$$U_a(\theta) = \sum_{i=1}^{k} \sum_{j=1}^{n_i} \frac{Y_{ij} - f(x_i, \theta)}{f(x_i, \theta)} \frac{\partial f}{\partial \theta_a}(x_i, \theta). \qquad (7.19)$$

For calculating the maximum likelihood estimator of θ, we will use the quasi-likelihood method, as in the binomial and multinomial models. In the case of overdispersion, the parameters σ^2 and τ of the variance function have to be estimated. We will use the quasi-likelihood method explained in Section 3.3.2. These methods are illustrated in the following cortisol example.

The methods for testing hypotheses or calculating confidence intervals for Poisson models are similar to those described in Section 3.4 for heteroscedastic nonlinear models and are not detailed here.

7.2.3 Cortisol Assay Example: The Poisson Nonlinear Model

First we consider a Poisson nonlinear model where the observations Y_{ij}, $j = 1, \ldots, n_i$, $i = 1, \ldots, 15$, have their expectation and their variance equal to $f(x_i, \theta)$ given by Equation (7.17).

Method The parameters are estimated by minimizing the deviance $D(\theta)$ (see Equation (7.18)).

Results

Parameters	Estimated Values	Standard Error
θ_1	133.78	5.61
θ_2	2760.3	23.8
θ_3	3.1311	0.244
θ_4	3.2188	0.151
θ_5	0.6218	0.049

The graphic of the standardized residuals presented in Figure 7.5 clearly shows that the dispersion of the residuals varies with the values of the fitted response.

Modeling the Variance Function We consider the case where the variance function is proportional to the variance of a Poisson variable: $\mathrm{Var}(Y_{ij}) = \sigma^2 f^\tau(x_i, \theta)$.

Method The parameters θ and τ are estimated using the quasi-likelihood method described in Section 3.3.2.

Results

Parameters	Estimated Values	Standard Error
θ_1	133.49	1.69
θ_2	2757.8	28.2
θ_3	3.2078	0.223
θ_4	3.2673	0.163
θ_5	0.6072	0.041
τ	2.1424	0.026
σ^2	0.0003243	

The graph of the standardized residuals presented in Figure 7.6 does not suggest any model misspecification. Therefore this is the preferred model, taking into account the overdispersion in the variance function, rather than the Poisson model. Finally, let us remark that the estimated standard errors of the parameters occurring in the regression function are modified when we take into account the overdispersion of the data.

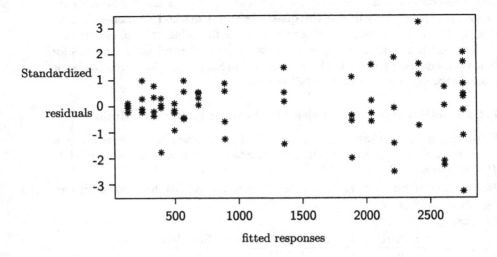

Figure 7.5. Cortisol assay: Standardized residuals versus fitted values under the Poisson model

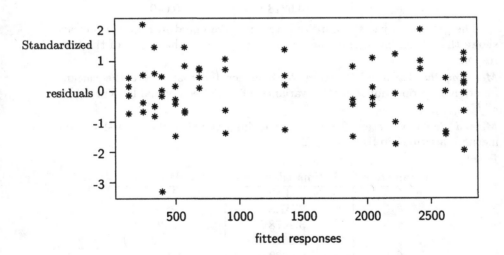

Figure 7.6. Cortisol assay: Standardized residuals versus fitted values under heteroscedasticity

7.2.4 Using nls2

We describe the Poisson model in a file called `corti.mpois`:

```
% file corti.mpois
% poisson regression model
resp cpm;
var v;
varind dose;
parresp n,d,a,b,g;
pbisresp minf,pinf;
subroutine;
begin
cpm= if dose <= minf then d else
        if dose >= pinf then n else
        n+(d-n)*exp(-g*log(1+exp(a+b*log10(dose))))
    fi fi;
v = cpm;
end
```

The data are stored in a *data frame* `corti`. We call `nls2` using its arguments as follows:

- The argument `method`—because minimizing the deviance $D(\theta)$ is equivalent to solving the quasi-likelihood equations defined by Equations (7.18), we will use `nls2` by setting the argument `method` to the value `"QLT"`.
- The argument `stat.ctx`—we have to use the components `sigma2.type` and `sigma2` of the argument `stat.ctx` that describes the statistical context of the analysis. By setting `sigma2.type` to the value `"KNOWN"` and `sigma2` to the value 1, we specify that σ^2 is known and equal to 1. Therefore σ^2 will not be estimated by the residual variance but will stay fixed to the value 1 throughout the estimation process.
  Moreover, calculation of the maximum likelihood, the minimum deviance, and the deviance residuals will be done only if the component `family` is set to the value `"poisson"`.

The starting values are set equal to the estimated values obtained with the nonlinear heteroscedastic regression model; they have been stored in the structure `corti.nl6` (see page 123):

```
> ctx <- list( theta.start=corti.nl6$theta,
                sigma2.type="KNOWN", sigma2=1)
> model <- list(file="corti.mpois", gamf=c(0,10))
> corti.nlpois <- nls2(corti, model,ctx, method="QLT",
                       family="poisson")
```

Then we display the result of the estimation process:

```
> cat( "Result of the estimation process:\n ")
> print(summary(corti.nlpois))
```

We plot the standardized residuals versus the fitted values of the response using the function plres.

Modeling the Variance Function as a Power of the Mean

The model is described in a file called corti.mpois2:

```
% file corti.mpois2
% overdispersion : one parameter tau
resp cpm;
var v;
varind dose;
parresp n,d,a,b,g;
pbisresp minf,pinf;
parvar tau;
subroutine;
begin
cpm= if dose <= minf then d else
     if dose >= pinf then n else
     n+(d-n)*exp(-g*log(1+exp(a+b*log10(dose))))
   fi fi;
v = exp(tau*log(cpm));
end
```

Then we call nls2 using its arguments as follows:

- The argument method—the parameters θ and τ are estimated by solving the quasi-likelihood equations defined in Section 3.3.2. nls2 is used by setting the argument method to the value "QLTB".
- Because σ^2 is an unknown parameter that has to be estimated, the components sigma2.type and sigma2 of the argument stat.ctx are set to their default values.

The estimated parameters and their standard errors are displayed:

```
> ctx <- list( theta.start=corti.nl6$theta,
               beta.start=1, max.iters=500)
> model <- list(file="corti.mpois2",gamf=c(0,10))
> corti.nlpois2 <- nls2(corti,model,ctx,method="QLTB")
> cat( "Result of the estimation process:\n ")
> print(summary(corti.nlpois2))
```

We plot the standardized residuals versus the fitted values of the response using the function plres.

References

[AAFH89] M. Aitkin, D. Anderson, B. Francis, and J. Hinde. *Statistical Modelling in GLIM*. Oxford Science Publications, New York, 1989.

[BB89] H. Bunke and O. Bunke. Nonlinear regression, functional relations and robust methods analysis and its applications. In O. Bunke, editor, *Statistical Methods of Model Building*, volume 2. Wiley, New York, 1989.

[BH94] A. Bouvier and S. Huet. nls2: Non-linear regression by S-Plus functions. *Computational Statistics and Data Analysis*, 18:187–90, 1994.

[BS88] S.L. Beal and L.B. Sheiner. Heteroscedastic nonlinear regression. *Technometrics*, 30:327–38, 1988.

[Bun90] O. Bunke. Estimating the accuracy of estimators under regression models. Technical report, Humboldt University, Berlin, 1990.

[BW88] D.M. Bates and D.G. Watts. *Nonlinear Regression Analysis and Its Applications*. Wiley, New York, 1988.

[Car60] N.L. Carr. Kinetics of catalytic isomerization of n-pentane. *Industrial and Engineering Chemistry*, 52:391–96, 1960.

[CH92] J.M. Chambers and T.J. Hastie. *Statistical Models in S*. Wadsworth & Brooks, California, 1992.

[Col91] D. Collett. *Modelling Binary Data*. Chapman and Hall, London, 1991.

[CR88] R.J. Carroll and D. Ruppert. *Transformation and Weighting in Regression*. Chapman and Hall, London, 1988.

[Cro78] M.J. Crowder. Beta-binomial anova for proportions. *Applied Statistics*, 27:34–7, 1978.

[CY92] C. Chabanet and M. Yvon. Prediction of peptide retention time in reversed-phase high-performance liquid chromatography. *Journal of Chromatography*, 599:211–25, 1992.

[Dob90] A.J. Dobson. *An Introduction to Generalized Linear Models*. Chapman and Hall, London, 1990.

[FH97] V.V. Fedorov and P. Hackl. *Model-Oriented Design of Experiments*. Springer, New York, 1997.

[Fin78] D.J. Finney. *Statistical Method in Biological Assay*. Griffin, London, 1978.

[FM88] R. Faivre and J. Masle. Modeling potential growth of tillers in winter wheat. *Acta Œcologica, Œcol. Gener.*, 9:179–96, 1988.

[Gal87] A.R. Gallant. *Nonlinear Statistical Models*. Wiley, New York, 1987.

[GHJ93]   M.A. Gruet, S. Huet, and E. Jolivet. Practical use of bootstrap in regression. In W. Härdle and L. Simar, editors, *Computer Intensive Methods in Statistics*, pages 150–66, Heidelberg, 1993. Physica-Verlag.

[GJ94]   M.A. Gruet and E. Jolivet. Calibration with a nonlinear standard curve: How to do it? *Computational Statistics*, 9:249–76, 1994.

[Gla80]   C.A. Glasbey. Nonlinear regression with autoregressive time-series errors. *Biometrics*, 36:135–40, 1980.

[Hew74]   P.S. Hewlett. Time from dosage death in beetles *Tribolium castaneum*, treated with pyrethrins or ddt, and its bearing on dose-mortality relations. *Journal of Stored Product Research*, 10:27–41, 1974.

[HJM89]   S. Huet, E. Jolivet, and A. Messéan. Some simulations results about confidence intervals and bootstrap methods in nonlinear regression. *Statistics*, 21:369–432, 1989.

[HJM91]   S. Huet, E. Jolivet, and A. Messéan. *La Régression Non-Linéaire: Méthodes et Applications à la Biologie*. INRA, Paris, 1991.

[HLV87]   S. Huet, J. Laporte, and J.F. Vautherot. Statistical methods for the comparison of antibody levels in serums assayed by enzyme linked immuno sorbent assay. *Biométrie-Praximétrie*, 28:61–80, 1987.

[LGR94]   F. Legal, P. Gasqui, and J.P. Renard. Differential osmotic behaviour of mammalian oocytes before and after maturation: A quantitative analysis using goat oocytes as a model. *Cryobiology*, 31:154–70, 1994.

[Liu88]   R. Liu. Bootstrap procedures under some non-i.i.d. models. *The Annals of Statistics*, 16:1696–708, 1988.

[LM82]   J.D. Lebreton and C. Millier. *Modèles Dynamiques Déterministes en Biologie*. Masson, Paris, 1982.

[McC80]   P. McCullagh. Regression models for ordinal data. *J. R. Statist. Soc. B*, 42:109–42, 1980.

[MN89]   P. McCullagh and J.A. Nelder. *Generalized Linear Models, 2nd edition*. Chapman and Hall, London, 1989.

[Mor92]   B.J.T. Morgan. *Analysis of Quantal Response Data*. Chapman and Hall, London, 1992.

[Pre81]   D. Pregibon. Logistic regression diagnostics. *The Annals of Statistics*, 9:705–24, 1981.

[Rat83]   D.A. Ratkowsky. *Nonlinear Regression Modeling*. M. Dekker, New York, 1983.

[Rat89]   D.A. Ratkowsky. *Handbook of Nonlinear Regression Models*. M. Dekker, New York, 1989.

[Ros90]   G.J.S. Ross. *Nonlinear Estimation*. Springer-Verlag, New York, 1990.

[RP88]   A. Racine-Poon. A Bayesian approach to nonlinear calibration problems. *Journal of the American Statistical Association*, 83:650–56, 1988.

[SW89]   G.A.F. Seber and C.J. Wild. *Nonlinear Regression*. Wiley, New York, 1989.

[TP90]   F. Tardieu and S. Pellerin. Trajectory of the nodal roots of maize in fields with low mechanical constraints. *Plant and Soil*, 124:39–45, 1990.

[VR94]   W.N. Venables and B.D. Ripley. *Modern Applied Statistics with S-Plus*. Springer-Verlag, New York, 1994.

[WD84]   H. White and I. Domowitz. Nonlinear regression with nonindependent observations. *Econometrica*, 52:143–61, 1984.

[Wil75]   D.A. Williams. The analysis of binary responses from toxicological exper-
           iments involving reproduction and teratogenicity. *Biometrics*, 31:949–52,
           1975.

[Wil82]   D.A. Williams. Extra-binomial variation in logistic linear models. *Applied
           Statistics*, 31:144–8, 1982.

[Wu86]   C.F.J. Wu. Jackknife, bootstrap and other resampling methods in regres-
           sion analysis (with discussion). *The Annals of Statistics*, 14:1291–380,
           1986.

Index

adjusted response curve 13
asymptotic level 32, 70

binomial model 153
bootstrap 35, 71
  B sample 36
  calibration interval 139
  confidence interval 36, 72, 165
  estimation of the bias 37
  estimation of the mean
    square error 37
  estimation of the median 37
  estimation of the variance 37
  heterogeneous variances 71
  prediction interval 138
  wild bootstrap 72

calibration 2, 135
confidence interval 32
  calibration interval 139, 142
  prediction interval 137, 138
  transformation of 33
  using the deviance 166, 207
  using the likelihood ratio test 73, 140,
    166, 207
  using the percentiles of a
    Gaussian variable 32, 72, 137, 139,
    206
    Student variable 32
  using bootstrap 36, 72, 138, 139, 165
confidence region 42, 72, 73
  confidence ellipsoids 43
  likelihood contours 43
  using the deviance 166

using the likelihood ratio test 73, 166
using the Wald test 73
covariance matrix 31
coverage probability 32
cumulative probabilities 202
cumulative residuals 212
curve comparison 35, 174

deviance 163, 204, 222
  residuals 168
  test 165, 207

empirical variance 5, 37
error 11
  correlations in 103
  independency 94
estimator
  least squares 11, 69
  maximum likelihood 12, 66, 162, 204,
    222
  minimum deviance 163, 204, 222
  quasi likelihood 67, 163, 164, 204, 222
  three-step alternate mean
    squares 69
  weighted least squares 13
experimental design 107

fitted values 94

Gaussian (observations, errors) 12, 66
goodness-of-fit test 111, 167, 215

heterogeneous variance 12, 61, 141
heteroscedastic model 61, 139, 161

Springer Series in Statistics

(continued from p. ii)

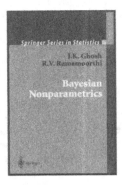
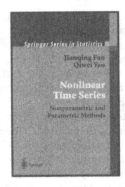
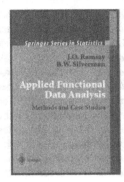
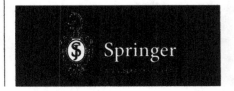